THE LAZY GUIDE TO HAPPY

THE LAZY GUIDE TO HAPPY

BEV CRIPPS

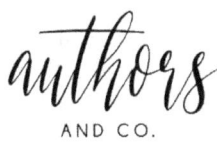

First published in Great Britain in 2023
by Authors & Co.
www.authorsandco.pub

Copyright © Bev Cripps 2023

Bev Cripps asserts the moral right to be identified as the author of this work in accordance with the Copyright, Designs and Patents Act 1988.

ISBN 978-1-915771-36-0 (paperback)
ISBN 978-1-915771-37-7 (hardback)

All rights reserved. No part of this book may be reproduced or transmitted in any form or by any means, electronic or mechanical, including photocopying, recording, or by any information storage and retrieval system without the written permission of the author, except where permitted by law or for the use of brief quotations in a book review.

Disclaimer
This book is intended to be a helpful guide on the topics discussed. It is not written as a diagnostic tool or a treatment for any condition. Please be sure to consult a medical practitioner before you make any decisions that may affect your health, particularly before you want to take part in any of the audio exercises. This is the author's own interpretation of positive psychology and resilience and her own adaptations of the various interventions and tools.

For Dot and John who gave me everything and told me I could be anything I wanted to be as long as I was happy.

CONTENTS

Introduction ... ix

1. What is happy and how do you get there? ... 1
2. Positive Emotions – the fabulous forty percent ... 10
3. Engagement – go with the flow ... 30
4. Relationships ... 47
5. Meaning and Purpose – why meaning matters and why we all need to matter ... 62
6. Accomplishment – being a goal-getter ... 79
7. Health Pillar ... 94
8. Resilience or how to ground yourself when the ground around you is moving ... 111

Now and Next ... 125
Notes ... 127
Acknowledgments ... 131
About the Author ... 135
Connect with me ... 137

INTRODUCTION

"I don't want to get to the end of my life and find I lived the length of it. I want to have lived the width of it as well."

— DIANE ACKERMAN

I know you are not lazy… far from it, in fact. The title of this book is intended to let you know that there are some low-effort things you can do which will help you on the path to *happy*. Contrary to what you may have read, you do not have to work very hard to build happiness in your day-to-day life. If you are time-poor, with a family, a career and financial responsibilities, you just can't hack *another* long list of things to add to your *already* long list of things to do. This book gives you low-effort, high-impact solutions that you can weave into your life to provide you with a baseline for happiness. You can be the busy person you are *and* expand your life for the better both for you and yours.

Perhaps you think (as I did) that 'happy' is the preserve of those with the time and finances to spend their days working on themselves. It might take the dedication of a yogi and the discipline of a drill sergeant to put in place all those things popular culture tells us we need to become happy, healthy, and to live our 'best lives'. Set this against the background of being offered a dream of happiness that will come when you have the right income level, the right job, the right size body. The concept of *I'll be happy when...* filters into our daily lives and happiness. It seems almost mythical – a nice to have. We barely have time to think about it and we are just too busy keeping everything on an even(ish) keel.

Happiness is, in fact, an inside job. It comes from within. We all have the potential to be happy and fulfilled. This book can start you on the path to a baseline that will elevate you above the 'just coping' mode you are in at the moment and set you on a path to *happy*. It may – and I don't want to alarm you unduly here – make you want to do more!

If your career is going well, you are turning up and you are coping, you may believe that's the measure of success. Perhaps you haven't noticed the slow leaks around you in the other areas of your life that this way of living is causing. I know some of you feel that you are keeping things going, yet when they all finally start to come together along comes another world event to set you back again.

I know some of you look to the casual observer as though it's all going well: you have the family and the successful job. Yet you experience an empty feeling as you work harder to maintain all this and wonder if this is really what it's all about. It might be that you wake up every day with a low level of anxiety, eyes firmly fixed on just getting through this week or waiting for that fortnight off far in the distance, knowing that if one more thing comes along it will derail everything. You'll be telling people you are fine but inside you've given up and are just trudging through. You are removed and disconnected.

You might feel borderline exhausted, disenchanted, overwhelmed and disappointed, but you soldier on for your family because what else is there to do?

You don't need me to tell you that things we have been sold which demonstrate a happy life – money, a great car, a successful career – don't make us happy. We pursue things we are told will make us happy. We say, *I'll be happy when...* I get the promotion, I have the new car, I get the relationship of my dreams. We always say, *I'll be happy when*. When you've tried to take another path, you've been put off. You are told you need to work hard and dial down on the things that will bring you a happy life.

I offer an alternative which fits into your busy life. It is another approach. You already have within you all you need to have a happy life. I would like to help you unlock the happy again by introducing you to low-effort, high-impact, zero-cost tools, based on evidence, that you can fit into your busy life. You can use them to build a baseline that will raise your happiness levels, increase your wellbeing, and improve the lives of those around you.

This book won't save your life but it may change it greatly for the better. It will describe the why and the how of building a happier and more resilient future and will give you low-effort zero-cost tools that have been scientifically tested to slot easily into your everyday life and routine.

The more I researched, the more I realised that awareness is fundamental. It is gold to just know there are things out there that can raise your levels of happiness if you do them regularly... and you don't have to get up at five in the morning to fit them into your day. If you are up that early, though, do give me a shout: I've always been a fully paid-up member of the wide-awake club.

Based on the principles of the science of positive psychology and resilience, chapter by chapter this book will take you through all the pillars proven to support a happy life. You will understand how they will build the foundations of a happy life both in their own way and taken together. We all have forty percent agency over our ability to be happy and experience positive emotions, regardless of our biology or what the world throws at us. With that most hopeful of statistics, you can follow the pillars and choose from the selection of low-effort, high-impact tools (or 'interventions' as they are known) and implement them during your busy day with no financial or time cost.

My 'journey' to *happy*, as happens sometimes, came out of some of the darkest and most stressful times of my life. But something in me always wanted something good, creative or, dare I say, life-affirming to come out of these events. The more I read, the more I realised that it is through darkness and stress that a lot of people come to find resilience and lead a happy life.

I first realised that my life was a little out of kilter a few years ago. One winter I was in the middle of prosecuting one of three murder trials which were listed one after another. My partner was a serving soldier in Afghanistan, during the winter that turned out to be one of the worst in an already awful conflict. Back in Wales, my father, who suffered from heart disease, was particularly unwell and I was spending a lot of weekends travelling to see him. One of my closest friends had recently been diagnosed with terminal cancer.

I visited my GP, not because of any of the above, but because someone had driven into the back of me. When you are really up against it, it always seems to be the way of things that one *extra* thing happens. While I was there, I mentioned I was having trouble sleeping. The doctor asked me if anything stressful was happening that may be keeping me awake. I told him all of the above and saw his eyes widen as the list went on. I reassured him that I was 'fine' and joked that I was saving my breakdown for the Christmas break. He rallied and suggested I should slow down a bit but since that wasn't a particular option for me at the time I battled on and, of course, it wasn't even Christmas yet …

I would love to say after the revelation of seeing through another person's eyes how manic my life had become that I became an immediate convert to all that I want to share with you. But as so often happens, life got in the way. It took two other significant moments before it finally clicked and I began to create my own positive, instinctive set of behaviours that turned out to be replicated in science and the evidence-based work that I now do... but more of that later.

As you expand into *happier* you at first see the quality of your life change imperceptibly for the better and then go on getting better in leaps and bounds. It turns out that the happier you are, the more successful you become, and the happiness levels of those around you will also increase. Your health, fitness and longevity improve. All these life-changing things happen because you feel better: you become more contented, more peaceful and even joyful.

These tools have been the bedrock of my last few years and enabled me to have a fresh perspective even when things do not go as planned. 'It' is always going to happen but these tools will help you build a strong core, enjoy life and ground yourself when the ground around you is moving. You will no longer feel like a victim of life events but more confident and with agency and control over yourself.

By profession, I am a criminal barrister and have been for *(ahem)* quite some time. I am also a clinical hypnotherapist, positive psychology coach, and resilience trainer qualified in NLP. I came to my more recent identities increasingly frustrated that, through no fault of their own, people I came across in the justice system had had their lives blighted for years by things totally outside their control.

I am a proponent of traditional therapy but I wanted to look for modalities that could change patterns and behaviours quickly. I tend to ask a lot of questions, which comes with the job. The question I asked myself in this case was how could these people deal with these events and go on to thrive and lead successful lives if that's what they wanted to do. It turned out there was a whole science of positive psychology and resilience which explored the basis of fostering growth, wellbeing and happiness whatever your circumstances.

I was hooked, not only because of the amazing results I saw from its implementation, but because it is evidence-based and rigorously tested. Hypnotherapy – also evidence-based – unlocks the key to the subconscious which itself is your most powerful ally in making a change. I can't promise that this book will save your life: I do know that if you implement even *some* of these tools into your everyday life, the evidence shows that things – and you – can only get better. After all, it can't hurt and it just might help you get *happy*.

1

WHAT IS HAPPY AND HOW DO YOU GET THERE?

"The more you strive and look for happiness the more you overlook the possibility that it is here already."

— ROBERT HOLDEN

"Happiness can be defined as an enduring state of mind consisting not only of feelings of joy, contentment and other positive emotions but also a sense that one's life is meaningful and valued."[1]

That may seem a very long way from where you are at the moment, but if you break this down, you'll see that we don't have to live on the level of constant joy and contentment but instead have it as a baseline in our lives. It is possible for us to increase our levels of happiness by being aware of the components of what has been discovered to be the basis of a happy life and by taking a look at them. You'd invest a little time in something this easy in order to feel better, wouldn't you?

We often think that happiness comes as a result of success but the truth is in fact the opposite. The journey to *happy* expands all areas of your life and impacts those around you.

Unlike the general knowledge we all have about how to be healthy, whether we implement that knowledge or not… you know, eat the right things, get outside and do your steps, drink more water and less alcohol… there doesn't seem to be the same basic understanding when it comes to our minds. I am definitely not the first person to say this should be taught in schools so that we have a great basis from which to start and go out and live happy, successful lives. Who knows, training the mind could become as mainstream as the idea that we should go the gym or do ten thousand steps every day. It involves a lot less physical effort and is extremely good for you.

Being a resilience trainer and twice certified coach in positive psychology, I have developed a coaching system around the core of these pillars that make a happy life. It utilises the power of the subconscious mind through hypnotherapy, NLP or eyes-closed change work (as the client prefers) to deal with anything that is holding them back, to help them with mindset and to reinforce the tools in each of the pillars. As you read the chapters you will find audios to help you use your subconscious on the path to *happy* in a way that is appropriate. Most of the audios do not use hypnosis though there is a short piece if you want to try.

All the audios can be accessed via my website found at the back of the book.

HOW DID THIS SCIENCE ALL BEGIN?

These components or pillars are the basis of the science of positive psychology. Its founder, eminent psychologist Martin Seligman, wanted to find an alternative to looking to the past to treat trauma and to understand how people could thrive and grow notwithstanding their experiences. It is a developing science which was trialled in its early days by the military. The tools (or interventions, as they are also called) we are going to come to have been used by the toughest of the tough and found to be effective and valuable so you may find them useful too.

The science of positive psychology is rigorously tested and evidence-based. I emphasise this because there's a lot here that some of you may perceive as 'woo'. I want to let you know that everything I suggest for you has been tested and successfully trialled by the most evidently 'anti-woo'.

From a vast study, Seligman identifies the six pillars that support wellbeing and a happy life. Those are: positive emotions, engagement, relationships, meaning, accomplishment and health.

We'll take a deep dive into those through the course of this book but it may be useful to know how you are at the outset in relation to these pillars. When I work with a coaching client, we start with this free survey which can tell you where you are in relation to those pillars. The Permah survey has been described as the psychological version of a Fitbit (or any other wearable you favour).

It provides a benchmark from which your progress can be measured. If you're wondering how, you can improve your wellbeing and your ability to feel good and function effectively, this would be a good place to start. Or you could take it, think about the various results and then focus on one that you feel most drawn to or that needs a bit of help. There are proven methods to improve on each element: try the tools in that element for a while to see what improvements you can make.

If you don't want to do the survey then just follow the chapters or dip into them as you wish. Each of them contains tools that you can use to enhance your wellbeing and happiness.

Your time is limited, I know, which is why I have made these tools 'busy proof'. They need only take up a small part of your day. Perhaps five minutes is absolutely all you can give to this. Please do start, and you may find the time expands. You might also add other tools into your day. Any steps forward can only benefit you… start with a single step and continue. Allow the momentum to drive you forward.

The Permah survey can be found at:

www.permahsurvey.com[2]

WHERE ELSE CAN YOU GET HELP TO HARNESS THE POWER OF THE SUBCONSCIOUS MIND?

The subconscious mind is said to be thirty thousand times more powerful than the conscious mind. Think of an iceberg. As little as one-eighth of the iceberg is visible above the water line. [3] The bergy bit (yes, that's what I am calling the visible sea ice) represents the conscious mind. We live on the tip of that iceberg – it is not only cold and uncomfortable but we are highly likely to fall off.

The relationship of the conscious mind to the subconscious is a bit like being a passenger on a bus. We sit there on the way to our destination feeling in control, knowing where we are going and feeling confident in being a passenger. Except, of course, we are not in control, the driver of the bus is. The driver decides where we stop, who gets on and who gets off. We have the illusion of control over the journey but we are actually being driven by the subconscious which is using its own patterns and beliefs.

In very general terms, and with apologies to neuroscientists everywhere, the subconscious mind is always trying to protect you but its methods are often outdated and have long since outlived their initial usefulness. Engaging the subconscious mind to act wholly with you is a useful tool to acquire. Awareness that you can use it is a start.

I have always wanted to do things as quickly as I can – though *carefully* quickly. I realised in the early hours of one morning how we can all use the subconscious to our benefit when I was indulging my insomnia by having a quick scroll on my phone (obvious note here: do not do that; it is very bad for you).

I came across hypnotherapy as a solution to my failure to sleep and started to research it. My research led me to Ali Campbell (not the one from UB40) who is extremely well-known in this field and I got hypnosis with him. The effects were immediate and effective and I loved it. Some people have issues with hypnosis but I found it such a relief to be able to relax that much and have that time out. I liked it so much I 'bought the company' as the ancient ad would put it. I trained in hypnosis and NLP with Ali who later became my mentor.

WHAT IS HYPNOSIS AND WHY CAN YOU CONSIDER IT A TOOL TO HELP YOU?

Hypnosis has traditionally had a bad reputation stemming from the days of stage hypnosis where skilled showmen were able to pick out highly suggestible people from an audience and put them into a trance for entertainment – burly guys acting like ballerinas… you know the drill.

Hypnosis is actually highly focused attention. Dr David Spiegel of Stanford University describes it as akin to looking through the telephotographic lens of a camera: you can see things in great detail but it is devoid of context. I cite Dr Spiegel here because not only has he one of the best voices in hypnotherapy, but he is a leading world expert in the field. He is a researcher and clinician and runs a clinic testing the efficacy of hypnotherapy. When we are looking at evidence-based tools to effect change quickly you can be sure that hypnosis is rigorously tested.

One of the greatest objections to hypnotherapy apart from that of religion is that the person is not in control. I would suggest the truth is quite to the contrary; a good hypnotherapist works *with* the client to achieve the desired result.

There are certain people who cannot be hypnotised. However, that is not to say that those who maintain they can't are not capable of being hypnotised if they want to be. Despite this, it is nigh impossible to hypnotise someone who does not want to be. We are not in fact losing control when we are hypnotised but *gaining* control over our minds. Hypnosis can show us that our brains have control over things in our bodies that we had no idea about, which is extremely valuable when we are talking about change.

In a study conducted by Doctor Spiegel, MRIs were used to monitor what happened to the part of the brain that controls the body (the insular). The subjects were put into hypnosis and told that they were going on a gastronomic trip in which they would be eating all their favourite foods prepared by the best chefs. As they continued this imaginary tour with imaginary food the level of their gastric acid secretion was measured at 87 percent. One woman under hypnosis asked to stop the experiment as she was full. When the participants were relaxed and talked about anything apart from food and drink, their secretions went down to forty percent and then settled at a baseline of 19 percent. The participants had not been given anything to eat.

Actually, the truth of the matter is that we spend a lot of our time in trance. If you become engrossed in a film you start to experience it and move away from its evaluation. Watching a horror movie, your body becomes tense as she walks down that alleyway. You clench your hands and your heart rate rises and a noise from outside makes you jump out of your skin: it's a door slamming. You get the idea. You are perfectly safe on your sofa.

ANOTHER TOOL IN THE KIT: NEURO LINGUISTIC PROGRAMMING.

In the interests of making a full disclosure, this is not a rigorously studied scientific modality. It did, however, have its beginnings in Santa Cruz, California in the 1970s where Professor John Grinder and his student Dr Richard Bandler wanted to develop models of behaviour to understand why some people achieved excellence in what they did and others found the same tasks very challenging or nigh on possible to achieve. I was drawn to it firstly because it appeals to my love of language and communication as a tool for change but also because it can work so quickly to change deep-seated patterns, behaviours, phobias and mindset. It is really impressive. It is a bit like humour in one sense: there are no definitive studies or research on what makes something funny yet we all know what makes us laugh.

Dictionary definitions of NLP include, "a model of interpersonal communication chiefly concerned with the relationship between successful patterns of behaviour and the subject experiences i.e., patterns of thought underlying them" and "a system of alternative therapy based on this which seeks to educate people in self-awareness and effective communication and change their patterns of mental and emotional behaviour."

One of the most powerful methods for change that I have had the good fortune to experience comes from NLP. I use it with all my clients who all report its powerful effects on them. Later in this book, we will look at harnessing the power of purpose in your life and you can experience NLP there too.

If you would like a short demonstration of what it can do for you on a surface level, please use the audio[4] and see how you get on.

Having established where you are now, let's see where you can get. You know… "Kid... you can move mountains." (*Dr Seuss*)

2

POSITIVE EMOTIONS – THE FABULOUS FORTY PERCENT

"So, the first step in seeking happiness is learning. We first have to learn how negative emotions and behaviours are harmful to us and how positive emotions are helpful."

— DALAI LAMA

One of the most exciting and hopeful discoveries I made when completing my coaching was that we have forty percent agency over our own happiness. Biology accounts for fifty percent and life circumstances for ten percent, but the rest we can influence ourselves!

HOW DID WE GET TO THIS?

Perhaps one of the reasons we think we can't change our essential levels of happiness is that we hold the view that that is just what we are like. There's Pollyanna on one end of the scale and Eeyore on the other and for the most part you can't change your place on the scale.

The nature or nurture debate had raged for years. One side argues that you are who you are and that's it. The chance of your genetics leads you to a life of Pollyanna or Eeyore or even much worse. Against that is the argument that you are the product of your upbringing and your circumstances define who you are. Again, you cannot change this. It is, as they say, what it is.

There is a third way. Neuroscience is now able to inform us that we can change our 'wiring' through neuroplasticity. However, let us begin with the more traditional question of nature or nurture.

Through my day job, I have met a number of eminent psychiatrists who have reported on participants in court cases. Over the years we have had time waiting at court when I've been able to ask them their views on the subject. I was intrigued to know how I was made up. I have a particular interest in this as I was adopted as a baby. I could see some traits of both my adoptive parents but wondered how much of me came from my genetics. I was introduced to the twin studies which were fascinating to me. Time and time again it was shown that twins who had been reared separately had the same characteristics as each other. There were remarkable similarities: being called the same name, looking alike, smoking the same brand of cigarette, marrying women of the same name, divorcing and then marrying women of the same name again… astonishing. This also led me to discover, as an adoptee, that my genetic make-up informed whether I was naturally optimistic or pessimistic. This made sense to me as my brother and I (both adopted) have diametrically opposite ways of looking at the world.

So yes, elements of both nature and nurture make us the "happy" people we are, but perhaps to a lesser degree than you think.

You may say that surely your level of *happy* depends a lot on what is happening around you. Back in the day, while some minor world event was going on (minor in comparison to maelstrom of Covid / war / recession) I heard a pundit on the radio (I lived in my car on the M25 in those days) saying that notwithstanding what was happening in the world, it was we who had control over the way we thought and it was our decision to be happy. I must have been going through one of the many episodes which I now call my 'resilience building phase', as I remember pooh-poohing that idea wholeheartedly. How could there be control in such circumstances? It turned out, and not for the first time you'll all be shocked to hear, I was wrong.

Life circumstances only have a ten percent effect on whether we have positive emotions and you can be sure that this has been rigorously tested across continents and populations.

Money can't buy you happiness… it helps, but only to a limited extent. Globally, many of us have a sense that you can be as rich as Croesus but it won't make you happy. Maybe we have a sense of that in our lives: your salary goes up and yet there is no real long-term effect on how you feel, or you have an unexpected windfall but once the initial excitement is over it doesn't really move the needle for you. Studies have shown that highly paid executives living in LA are not substantially happier than the Amish who live simple lives away from all we are told are markers of success. Kolkata slum dwellers are happier than people who live in deprived parts of the US, who, while comparatively poor in USA terms, have a much better standard of living than the poor of India. Once a certain level of need has been fulfilled, it seems that money does not add to our happiness.

I am not pretending for a moment that living in the middle of a crisis caused by war or famine is part of this statistic. Of course, that is a time for basic survival.

We in the privileged nations have now experienced what it is like to be in the grip of an event that is not within our control, when everything we know is no longer as it was. Perhaps it has given us at least the beginning of an insight into the circumstances experienced by many people in the world. But we adapted, as we are coded to do. I am not taking away from those who worked and lived on the front line for us, but in the main the new 'normal' was established. A more reflective state of mind came upon some of us. Having been unable to do what we do, we started thinking more. It certainly came to my mind that for many of us, as long as everything looked all right and we were functioning in work, then we thought we must be fine. It didn't seem to matter before what the cost was to ourselves, our wellbeing or our families... but now it does.

THE VERY GOOD NEWS

Do we really have any agency over how we think and feel? Yes, we do. The very good news is that we have a whole forty percent agency over the positive emotions we generate and feel through our intentional activity. A forty percent chance to dial up our happiness notwithstanding our baseline and external events is huge. It was the first of many life-enhancing discoveries I made when I studied to become a 'pos psych' coach.

BROADEN AND BUILD

Positivity pioneer Barbara Fredrickson introduced the concept of *broaden and build*. By this method you can expand your positive emotions. I hope the benefits of doing that are obvious but it is deeper than just turning negative emotions into positive ones; positive emotions expand your mind, help your performance at work or in sports/hobbies in which you wish to excel, and enhance your overall wellbeing. But more than that, they help you build up reserves you can draw on in the bad times – or, when a great opportunity presents itself, you can take up the ball and run.

Essentially, you feel better. You feel more in control. A particularly lovely side effect is that this spreads to those around you when they begin to notice you seem a little, well... lighter. You will read a lot about the ripple effect as we go on and how it is a real, positive by-product of using your forty percent. By doing very little, the people around us are positively affected. That can't possibly be bad. Of course, as you love some of those people, it is a very good thing indeed.

THE HOW

Knowing about this is great, but how do you do it? There are myriad things you can do. Doing the ones, you enjoy most will clearly be most beneficial. I know you are busy so I have trialled them and I offer you a selection of low-effort, high-impact techniques that give you the most bang for your very busy buck and that you can incorporate seamlessly into your day.

Toxic positivity should get a mention here too. What we are doing is not about ignoring what happens and breezily continuing with everything. Toxic positivity is toxic as it encourages us to trample over our emotions and builds up trouble for us all.

THE LAZY GUIDE TOOLS TO ENHANCING YOUR POSITIVE EMOTIONS:

Some tools dial up the positive while others dial down the negative. You choose which tools to use. They will all increase your capacity for positive emotions.

DIALLING UP THE POSITIVE

Connect with nature. A low-effort method of enhancing your positive emotions is simply to get outside, preferably into nature, but anywhere outside is good enough. Enjoying where you are and taking time to appreciate what is around you can give you so many benefits. It is an obvious tool, but nevertheless, we sometimes take for granted what we have. It is easier when you have access to the sea (one of the joys of my life in all weathers, both growing up and now) or green spaces. But getting outside even in the most uninspiring places can give you that break you need. Even in a city, looking up can give you views of things you haven't seen before.

If you are an early riser, whether by nature or your insomnia insists on waking you up at God-awful-o'clock, you can get double the benefit of being outside. Try to get outside first thing in the morning for just ten minutes and expose yourself to natural sunshine or daylight, depending on the time of year. Natural light in your eyes at that time, without sunglasses (though do not stare directly at the sun), helps your circadian rhythm enormously and therefore helps your sleep, as well as the aforementioned benefits.

Gratitude. I know it has become almost a self-development cliché but it is no less valid for this. If you'll indulge me for a moment, I can explain how important this really is. The eminent Harvard psychiatrist Doctor Conti tells us that the two fundamentals of mental health are agency and, you've guessed it, gratitude.

Here we are dealing with how you develop agency in the forty percent so let's add to it this fundamental piece. Happily, for all of us who have no time, it takes only the smallest effort. It is barely there and you'll hardly notice doing it again and again.

Just in case you are cynical, heaven forbid, about its efficacy, you should know that much of this work was trialled in the US Army, not a population particularly known for their affection for things some would consider 'woo'.

Briefly, the founder of positive psychology, Martin Seligman, was asked to set up protocols that would foster post-traumatic growth to combat the ever-growing cases of PTSD in veterans and its tragic, worst-scenario consequences. Trialling these interventions in the army is a good vehicle for testing their efficacy. Firstly, there is very little opportunity for people to be nay-sayers since they are obliged to cooperate. Secondly, you are dealing with a population who in the main are quite stressed for a living. If it works for them, it can work for us. However tough you may be, you may not be quite as tough as, for example, a Navy Seal.

The exercise became known as *hunt the good stuff*. Sergeants were asked to record something good that had happened to them every day in the 'three blessings journal' and each day they shared what they had written down. It was feared that these NCOs would consider this intervention as psychobabble but across regiments this exercise received an anonymous 4.9/5 approval rate.

In one study, Seligman implemented this one happiness-enhancing strategy to a group of extremely depressed people on a psychiatric ward. Although many of this group had difficulty leaving their beds, they logged on to a website where they were asked to recall and write down three good things that had happened that day. Everyone managed it, recording things like a call they had received from a family member or that the sun had come out that day. This exercise lasted for fifteen days. After, the group's results were objectively tested and the majority went from, "severely depressed to mild to moderately depressed, 94 percent of them reporting they had experienced relief."[1] It is a very powerful tool.

Out of everything I've learned about positive psychology, **three good things** is my all-time favourite intervention. In our busy lives we often dwell on what happened that went wrong and often fail to see the good stuff. When I did my positive psychology coaching course, the first question asked every week was, "What went well for you this week? What gave you joy?" I used to struggle with that at times given the fact I was usually involved in a case whose content didn't lend itself to *happy*. But I quickly came to realise that this was exactly the sort of question that needed to be asked. Many of us get caught up in the 'doing' of life and ignore the other things happening around us.

Do this for yourself now...

Write down three good things that went well for you during the day and why they went well. Writing? I know you might not want to, but it is better if you can so that you have a record of them. It is so easy to forget the good things that happen to you when you go through the bad. But recording the good things can be a reminder for us. There will be bad days, of course, when the best you can do is say that you are above ground and breathing. I got that one from my father, one of the most resilient people I know. He suffered from significant health problems for years yet really lived life. On a not so drastic day you might say that it didn't rain today. The value in doing this even on a bad day is that you've gone through a very bad day yet you're here writing in this journal focusing on the good that happened in the day. The good can be as small as a smile from the person at your local coffee shop or as big as a bloody huge triumph in your life. Write those down too. Say why it went well and how you felt. We often let our achievements go; so many of us dismiss them.

I have a friend who wrote a Sunday Times bestseller. I first met her at a business event and she told us all about what she did and her background, which was impressive enough. At the end, she told us she had written a Sunday Times bestseller in a manner in which you might say, "I got first place in my son's school sack race." Everyone was immediately agog and wanted to know all about it. It was one of the first things, this lovely modest woman could have mentioned, yet didn't until prompted. I suggested that she get a tattoo on her wrist so that she would be reminded of it and I really hope she has!

You can return to this library of good things and remind yourself of them when things are not going so well. It can buoy you up and give you the confidence to seize an opportunity when you are given one.

For additional benefit, do this last thing at night before you go to sleep to make an end to whatever sort of day you have had and to put yourselves in the best possible condition for a good night's sleep.

This is a really lovely intervention to turn into a routine with your kids, and perhaps even with the truculent younger teenagers. With teen anxiety on the rise, this provides a little routine and an oasis for you to have special time with them. For the little ones, it encourages them to focus on the good that has happened in their day. For the teens... if drill sergeants can come to appreciate this intervention, even the mini cynics can come to enjoy this as a time for them, after they have made the obligatory 'Kevin' responses and made some grudging participation. It leaves them in a positive frame of mind before they sleep and it will for you too. The last thing the subconscious experiences before it goes to sleep is an emphasis on the positive.

Savouring – 10 X the good in things and dial up the positivity. Again, there is nothing to do here but be aware of what you experience. The way people approach good things happening to them is dependent on the person. There are those who know something good is coming so they plan to enjoy it, think about how it's going to be when they are there and then they enjoy the moment. There are others who think more negatively that it is too good to be true or have a sense of unease when the good thing happens, or disbelief that this is actually happening to them and feel that something is bound to go wrong. Even so, it is possible to increase the enjoyment of things and events. To savour these things and to really enjoy them, just take time to appreciate what is going on. It's not analysis, it's being actually in the moment.

Literally wake up and smell the coffee. The pandemic, if it did nothing else that was good, allowed us an opportunity to see what we have and to take joy in the small things. I remember one of the best days was when I was out for my allotted exercise time and saw my local coffee shop by the beach was open and serving takeaway coffee. I have never been so happy to stand in a queue, shout my socially distant order, pass the time of day with my friend the coffee shop manager, and then take my coffee onto the beach. I can still taste the coffee and I hadn't felt so in the moment and grateful in a very long time. Small things…

Freudenfreude: what a great word. It is the opposite of schadenfreude, meaning to find joy in another's success. Savour and share your successes. A lot of us are really bad at this. We quite happily detail the latest disasters and mistakes we make but dismiss the successes we have. Why not tell someone about this? You know the people who will be happy for you and happy to share in your success. Tell them how you feel and appreciate the acknowledgement so the positivity is dialled up for you both.

Be kind – or rather, selfishly unselfish. Let me explain. Being kind is an evidence-based, tested way to increase your own levels of happiness. Unsurprisingly, doing good things for those around you makes you happy and fulfilled so it is a complete win-win. Kindness to others is also kindness to ourselves.

A really great and useful example of the effectiveness of being kind (and how it may even save your life!) is the doctors' study.[2] Doctors were given a notional patient who suffered from liver disease. The researchers told them the patient's diagnosis (they were given a deliberately incorrect diagnosis) and they were asked to assist with the treatment. The doctors were split into groups: one group were given sweets by volunteers who spoke appreciatively to them as they discussed the diagnosis. The other group were left to themselves. Those who had received the sweets and the kind words were quickest to discover the wrong diagnosis and were also more creative, able to think of innovative kinds of treatment. Those who had not been treated kindly tended to follow the incorrect diagnosis or take longer to get to the fact it was incorrect. This study has been replicated with doctors at all levels of their career with similar results. The lesson is, next time you go to the doctor take a bag of sweets! You also might like to think about how you approach and talk to people to allow them to be at their best.

A nice low-effort kindness exercise is to do five kind things in a day as the opportunities present themselves to you. This also has a positive effect on those around you. It is the simple things that are really appreciated. Just exchanging a few words with someone can absolutely raise their day and the power of a smile can be immeasurable to someone in a desperate state.

Loving kindness meditation. I have included this short meditation for you[3]: all you have to do listen. Researchers have found that practising this for seven weeks significantly increased positive emotions which led to an increase in mindfulness, purpose and even a decrease in symptoms of illness. It is a powerful tool that you can very easily put into your day – maybe during the quiet time at the beginning of the day. Just give it a try and see how it makes you feel and then try it again and see how long you want to continue with it.

Just have fun. Do you remember years ago before the grind got you? You used to do things for the fun of it. You know what lights you up but these days, if you don't fit it into your schedule it doesn't happen. Perhaps you need to be a little less spontaneous than you used to be. Put fun things in your schedule and do them. At some point, a noise will startle you and you'll realise that it's you laughing, really laughing. I heartily suggest you do what you love (within the law, of course) and do it more often!

DIALLING DOWN THE NEGATIVITY – PUT YOURSELF IN A MORE POSITIVE STATE

Disconnect from noise. Don't be too shocked but in general this involves limiting any media time, especially first thing in the morning... sorry.

How many of us pick up our phones first thing? I think it's a rare person who doesn't or hasn't. I'm not anti-social media: it has had massive benefits and you can use it to enhance your forty percent – if you use it well.

However, recent studies show the average person spends two hours a day on the phone. You may say that's not so much and there's no reason why you shouldn't. Maybe you have thoughts like *I deserve it... I'm worn out.* Perhaps you say *I need to keep current with the news, the markets, the economy, the Real Housewives and what Noodles the Pooch is up to on Insta these days and what about those llamas?* (Ahem this might be me, by the way.)

You may have a point about those two hours, once in a while. *But...* an average of two hours every day is fourteen hours a week, fifty-six hours a month and 472 hours a year. This means you are giving up eight whole working days a month – three working months a year – to Messrs Zuckerburg and Musk. It is no wonder that we have no time. It reminds me of that quote from Aldous Huxley about the dictators of the future and how we would come to love them. (It is social media and media generally I'm referring to, not individuals.)

Take back your time and use it for you. Be aware, use media for good and for real entertainment. But mindless scrolling is like empty calories: it depletes us. Every time we look at a post our brains make decisions to like, not like, comment or move on. It really does go some way to explain how we are more frazzled than we used to be. I don't know if any of you have seen that *My life in weeks*[4] poster, a chart showing the 4,576 weeks of the average human life span. How you choose to spend them is up to you, but at least make that choice consciously. All of a sudden, the llamas aren't quite so funny.

If you want to dial down on that a little (pardon the pun) my clients and I have found a little delay in our phone activity first thing very effective.

I liken looking at your phone, email or social media at that time of the morning to having a group of people shouting at you when you've just woken up. Just having that time for yourself in the morning, even five minutes to yourself, can be gold. Be outside or just look outside. Have your tea. Read if you want to but nothing connected with work, and maybe jot some thoughts down. Have this little oasis for you. Whatever the day brings, at least you have started it from a position of calm.

The life-changing magic of a glass of water. Since you are up, do this one thing. Have a glass of water when you get out of bed, every day without fail, and acknowledge and congratulate yourself that you are doing it. I got this idea from Dr Nicole Perera's book *How to Do the Work*. In it, she describes how a patient, an MS sufferer who was about to be confined to a wheelchair, started this one thing every morning. However bad she felt, she was able to do that simple task. Her faithful adherence to it allowed her to gain certainty and hope that she was committed to something. Little by little, she built confidence in herself. What she was able to do expanded as did her strength.

Something this small can bring you back from the brink. I know this as I have seen it work successfully in my coaching practice. The CEO of an amazing and successful ethical company came to me exhausted. although he outwardly appeared 'fine and functioning'. He thought he had nothing left to give to coaching but saw it as a possible life raft to help.

After our first session of hypnotherapy, I suggested the morning glass of water and doing only that in addition to his usual responsibilities. I've still got the picture he sent, grinning and making a 'cheers' to the camera. It was the start of the turnaround and he understood it. It's not the water – though always drink lots – it's knowing there are very small things you can do, no matter what is happening around you, to be consistent and have the confidence to move on to other things and grow. Broaden and build in action.

So, a zero-effort intervention for you is no phone first thing in the morning. For something that needs a little more effort, give yourself a designated time to interact with it and do no more. If it gets too bad, put the phone in another room. At the very worst, lock it out of sight in the car.

MANAGE NEGATIVE THINKING MORE QUICKLY THAN YOU THINK

We have a bias towards negativity. The part of the brain that has followed us up out of the oceans (often described as the reptilian brain) is wired to the negative. It sees threats everywhere and causes those feelings of intense dread. It is a cliché but nonetheless true that we are still wired to run from the sabre tooth tiger, even though these days the response can be activated by a summons from the department head or by opening one of those brown envelopes that the UK tax people still like to send.

The negativity need not come from the inside. Turning on the news during the past couple of years means is not difficult for the mind to dial down into negative thoughts. I don't have to tell you that our thoughts often spiral and we begin to ruminate. Many of us unconsciously catastrophise and things become worse. Or rather, we think they do. *Thought* here is the operative word. Of course, we can be affected by truly horrendous events but even the mundane can build and get out of hand. We don't know where we are and everything is bleak – anxiety builds and we feel less confident. However, the news is good. We can stop the downward spiral and wind it back up. It takes an amazingly short time to do it.

Be a disruptor……

This way of thinking is especially good for all my lawyers out there and for all you lovely souls who enjoy a good… let's call it a *debate*. You are going to deploy those skills on your own behalf, going in to bat for you, taking up arms… you get the picture.

As is often the case, start with awareness:

1. Identify the thought or belief.
2. Externalise it. Imagine (or you may not have to) that this comes from a person who makes your life miserable.

3. Look for evidence that it is true. If someone said this to us, we would dispute it (or have many arguments with them in private which they didn't know about) to put them right. Because the thought comes from us, we tend to treat it as if written in stone. Why do we do this? We wouldn't take it from someone else so why do we accept it from ourselves? We do have a negativity bias but again this is something over which we have control.
4. Imagine a friend says this about themselves. What would you say to them to help? We also need to have this rebuttal reinforced so this is where you can become the investigator – is it true? Are you sure? In what ways is it not true? Is there another explanation? Is that thought actually based in reality? I wouldn't mind betting that on many occasions you'll find it's not.

If sometimes you find the evidence to back things up and things *are* as bad as you think, what then? Try not to catastrophise. Take a pause and ask what this really means in the future. Again, be aware. Think of times you or others have been in that situation. Is it changeable and what can you do to stop it? Has this situation or belief got any use at all for you? There is a space between stimulus and response[5] and being aware that there are options can reinforce that pause for you to be able to deal with these things a little better.

This process does not ask you to override your thoughts or feelings. Instead, it asks you to focus on them but in a different, healthier way. If you feel that you do want to acknowledge them without being a disruptor, by all means do, but try to set a specific amount of time for them and reward yourself when you keep to that allotted time.

You have now given yourself the gift of forty percent more agency and gratitude. I suggest that, with a little hope and a nod to the 1990s, things can only get better!

3

ENGAGEMENT – GO WITH THE FLOW

"Being at one with the music, time stopping and a loss of self-consciousness during an absorbing activity… in flow we merge with the object."

— MARTIN SELIGMAN

WHAT IS ENGAGEMENT AND WHY DO YOU NEED TO KNOW ABOUT IT?

Engagement is one of the pillars of positive psychology. It describes an effortless state that we are all familiar with. When we are in it, we can be said to be truly happy. It shows up when we are completely absorbed in what we are doing so that we have no sense of time passing and are completely unself-conscious. This is called the flow state, otherwise described as being *in the zone*. The beauty of this state is that it is unconscious and requires little effort. We all have been in that state but unless we are full-time composers or high-level athletes, we often don't recognise it for what it is. When we do register it, we do so with delight and then get right back into the 'doing of the things'.

THE BENEFITS OF BEING IN FLOW?

When you are really engaged, your sense of control over what you do is enhanced, your belief in yourself expands and your confidence levels rise. These benefits are out of all proportion in relation to the effort needed. There is a feeling of being more involved in life rather than the passenger on that bus, where life rushes past the window and your focus narrows to the list of obligations you have to fulfil. As our lives become busier and more chaotic, these flow experiences fade and we move away from these great opportunities to enhance our daily lives and to really live.

Remember a time when you were in flow, when you were completely absorbed in what you were doing, when you felt secure in your abilities and just how good you felt. You can actually expand those experiences so they become more a part of your life. As well as experiencing flow when you are doing something you love, "more often than not people experience flow at work".[1] Since you have to be there anyway, it wouldn't be the worst thing to have more of these experiences at work, would it?

Let's look at why this is important to your general wellbeing and happiness.

Research has shown that ninety percent of people are unaware of themselves and why they do what they do. Ten percent are strongly aware. By moving yourself over to the ten percent, you are already winning.

A good way to enhance your experiences of flow is to remove distractions. Some of you may suggest that you are in flow when you watch TV or play computer games and science agrees that for about eight percent of the time you are, but if you come away from those experiences feeling like you've overeaten, feel guilty or unhealthy then that's not being in flow. If TV is your hobby, great, but be mindful about what you want to watch and make it something challenging. Sharks, evading border control and speeding up the motorway are not what I'm talking about here (you know who you are). This is called the pursuit of obsessive pleasures. As the verbiage suggests, it is not great. We are after intrinsic pleasures instead.

Being in flow is an antidote to getting stuck in a negative state of worrying obsessively about what can go wrong.

What does it feel like to be in flow? It is when:

- The activity matches and challenges your level of skill. It should be just a bit above your skill set. If we can do things too easily this becomes a bit pedestrian and boring. As busy as we all are, as long as we are doing an activity we like, we are wired to enjoy a bit of a challenge.
- The activity has clear goals and immediate feedback. An athlete in flow has a goal to win the game/race

and feedback from spectators is immediate. Feedback is the way you feel good after the activity.
- You are completely concentrating on the activity. In general terms, our minds can deal with 110 bits of information a minute. If you are attempting to be in flow while doing something (writing a chapter of a book, for example), if someone is talking and you are listening in then that's sixty bits of your bandwidth gone; if someone starts talking to you, that's it – you've used up your bandwidth and your concentration is broken. In the state of flow, you are completely focused and absorbed. Nothing else is relevant.
- You experience oneness with the activity – you have no sense of anything else: you are in your own bubble.
- You experience a sense of calm and a loss of self-consciousness. So often in everyday life, we are conscious of how we appear. We can be anxious about what people think and get caught up in that. When you are in flow, all that is left behind and nothing else matters. You are giving all your bandwidth to the activity and that critical voice in your head is silenced. It stops monitoring and analysing all that you do.
- You lose track of time. This is a wonderful thing to experience. In the day-to-day, time can drag when you are doing those tasks that you have to do but find dull. Flow is the polar opposite to this and time just goes. Have you ever had the experience of being

so wrapped up in a book that you look up and are surprised that it is dark outside or realise that you are cold because the temperature has changed?
- You have a feeling of being in control. You are using your skills and your strengths to their best and being appropriately challenged.
- You feel that the activity is worth doing for its own sake. It is not forced. It gives you a sense of meaning and you feel an intrinsic reward. It is not dependent on external recognition.

REALLY GO WITH THE FLOW

Now we've broken down the flow state and thought about how good it feels, it may be good to know that you can create more of it in your life to expand the *happy*. You can even use these tools in the work arena for things you're not overly keen on.

THE LAZY GUIDE TOOLS FOR GOING WITH THE FLOW.

Some low-effort things for you to do: -

Put yourself into a flow state to remind you how it feels. Find a quiet place and pay attention to yourself for a few moments. If you need it, there's a short audio to help[2]. It may help you to write the experience down afterwards.

But for now, just think of a time when you experienced a sense of flow. What were you doing? When was it? What had you done to get into that flow state? How did you feel? Were you alone or were there other people around? What was the end result? How did you feel afterwards? Did you feel a sense of achievement? Did you feel like you were a capable person? Think about these things for a little while and savour those feelings.

With those feelings in mind, can you visualise / imagine a stronger future when you build more of this into your life, your home life, relationships and even work? We spend so much time at work... why not use your flow experience while you're there? You have a lot to gain, not least becoming a happier and more productive person.

TAP INTO YOUR STRENGTHS AND FIND YOUR SUPERPOWERS

A really good way to increase flow in your work and life is to learn about your strengths. Many of us are unaware of our strengths, never mind how to use them. They are a fabulous foundation for what you do in your life. When you know what they are and use them, you are more engaged and in flow. Knowing your strengths helps in all areas of your life: you perform better in your relationships and in work.

I love this positive approach to progressing our lives and happiness. Many of us come from a background that has encouraged us to focus on our weaknesses, to try hard to build them up so that what we can do better, while our strengths were barely praised. However, there is a strong body of research that suggests developing our strengths actually leads to our 'weaknesses' being improved too and coming up to meet our strengths. We tend to think that if we are good at something, that is the end of it and we do not think it needs to be developed. We focus on our weaknesses, and try to fix the weaknesses: this approach may prevent failure – but building on and expanding your strengths leads to success.

In case you need more convincing that this new approach is a far healthier and more successful way to get on in life, consider the words of General David Petraeus who broke the traditional training mode of the forces. He said, "The big idea… is to produce more post-traumatic growth… to approach training our soldiers' strengths rather than drilling their weaknesses out of them."

GETTING TO KNOW YOU

How do you know what your strengths are? This is another area where the ninety percent don't know the answer, but you can become one of the ten percent. You can very easily find out what they are, how to develop them and how to use them.

I use two indicators in my coaching practice: firstly, the Gallup Clifton Strengths Assessment and secondly, the Values in Action Survey (VIA). Gallup, a paid-for product. I mention it here as you may want to find out about them or suggest the survey at your workplace, perhaps as professional development.

I am really drawn to the VIA survey. It is a free survey based on Martin Seligman's huge cross-border study of values which are common to us all, regardless of race, culture, economics or class. There are six basic strengths which are then broken down into individual strengths. They are: wisdom and knowledge; transcendence; courage; humanity; temperance and justice.

It is really interesting to find out what your strengths are. Unlike talents, which tend to be innate, strengths can be developed, strengths are more badges of character. The survey can be found at www.viacharacter.org and will take five to ten minutes. You might find out something about yourself that you didn't know. Knowledge of yourself is power because once you know your strengths you can deploy them as your superpowers. All superpowers come with a bit of kryptonite to watch out for which we'll talk about later. For now, let's just take a deep dive into your strengths.

I will also show you how to deploy your strengths in relation to expanding your flow. Your flow state, remember, depends partly on your current level of skill being equal to or almost equal to the task.

My top five strengths on the VIA are Kindness, Humour, Creativity, Gratitude and Curiosity.

When you look at your list of strengths you may be more drawn to some than others. Some may resonate with you, while others feel dull. These are called selective strengths. You may not have realised that you had some strengths, or even not even recognised them *as* strengths. For example, my top Gallup strength is that I am strategic. Those who know me well and claim I have no practical bent might be surprised to hear that. I would not have ever described myself as strategic and yet, when I looked at what I do for a particular part of my profession, I realised that I was very strategic. It's something lawyers have to be good at or learn to be good at.

It is important not to look at strengths in isolation. Also remember that strengths that appear lower down the list are not weaknesses. The qualities listed lower down on your list will be qualities that are less dominant: this does not mean that you do not have those strengths.

You may not immediately identify with the strengths that come up, but sometimes that has a lot to do with the environment you're in, particularly if you've been there for a while and you are not happy. Simply focus on the strengths and you will see where they show up and perhaps get a sense of how you could use them better elsewhere.

What does an active knowledge and use of your strengths give you? Research shows that people who are aware of their strengths are six times happier and more engaged, and experience a 7.8 percent increase in productivity in the workplace. You're there anyway so you might as well benefit from it. The only effort it involves is being you!

I mentioned earlier that all superpowers come with their own kryptonite. Sometimes, overusing your strengths can be a weakness. For example, kindness is my top strength. When this gets out of whack, I find myself spreading myself too thin and becoming exhausted with no time left for me. I'm a high-energy girl, or rather, because of my sleep patterns I'm awake for a long time and have a low boredom threshold so I like doing lots of things, but sometimes it can get a bit much.

THE LAZY GUIDE TOOLS FOR BENEFITTING FROM YOUR STRENGTHS:

Take a look at what they are. Discover what strengths you have. Which strengths can you see that you use on a daily basis? You can, if they are up for it, do the survey with your significant other or friend. Most of us like finding things out about ourselves and who doesn't like a good quiz? Ask them what strengths they see in you and tell them what strengths you see in them. It helps foster your relationship. It is also great for reinforcing confidence so you could try it with older kids. It is a great key to know how to best encourage them, so far away from the bias towards talking about our weaknesses with which we were brought up.

Frame it till you make it. Use your imagination. It is said that our brains have difficulty telling the difference between what is real and what is imagined, so a great tool to enhance your strengths is to imagine what could happen if you used them to the full. Have positive images of what your future looks like when you use these strengths.

Put a daily reminder on your phone / in your journal (if you are one of my people) to use one particular strength on that day. In your morning quiet time, think of how you can enhance your day's tasks with it. Play a game with it. You can use your strengths in a novel way.

Try strengths journalling. If you're not into stationery, you can do this on your beloved phone to make it a little more palatable.

At the end of the day, review what went well and not so well. When you are thinking of something that went well, what part did you play in it, however small? Notice what strengths you used and how they came into play. This rebalances the negativity bias we all have.

When you become aware of tasks or activities that you are less keen on, start noticing what you don't like about them. In our ideal world, we wouldn't be doing anything that didn't appeal to us or that didn't play to our strengths; perhaps we wouldn't be working at all. In our real world, however, this thing called work takes up a large amount of our lives. Let's see if we can make it fun or rather, use our strengths to our best advantage, and see how it goes for us.

It's easy to think of flow experiences for a concert pianist or a surgeon, in which they become completely absorbed in their work... in flow. But what about other jobs in which, on the face of it, the opportunities for creativity are not overwhelming? We can find flow in all walks of life.

Martin Seligman tells a story about visiting a friend who had a terminal illness. He sat by his friend in the small hospital ward. A man who worked at the hospital was hanging some pictures on the wall, taking a great deal of care where each picture went, standing back and making sure that they were hung right. He engaged in conversation with Seligman and told him that he worked as a janitor at the hospital. Unasked, he told the father of positive psychology that he took great care with the paintings and from time to time would remove them and change them around so the patients would have something novel and pleasant to look at during their time on the ward. Seligman describes how he was watching flow in action. The man was doing something which was greater than himself and was completely unconscious of anything except the task in front of him.

A wider study of hospital janitors found a population who really enjoyed their work as well as those who said that they worked to support their families. Each group's reason for working was valid, of course, but the group who said they enjoyed their work were aware of their skills and strengths and felt that these were being used to the best value. They viewed themselves as having an essential role in assisting the doctors and nurses in their work by providing a safe, clean environment for the patients and had a determination to do something which would increase their comfort and value.

Closer to home, a younger member of my family is working a customer-facing job that is sometimes quite gruelling in order to fund her studies in psychology. Two of her top strengths are kindness and humour, and now that she is aware of these strengths, she focuses on those during her interactions with the less cheerful customers. She has told me how she has increased her enjoyment in her job by bringing a bit of sunshine into people's lives – even the ones who aren't quite so delighted with her sunny disposition!

Mindfulness to enhance engagement and get into flow. There is an old Zen saying: *"You should sit in meditation for twenty minutes every day unless you're too busy, in which case you should sit for an hour."*

You may be starting to notice that the essence of moving on in the world in this low-effort way involves you becoming aware of what you already possess within you. You don't have to seek it out or struggle to access it – just take the time to notice. When we seek to enhance our engagement, this issue of awareness is very important.

Mindfulness was first developed in the 1970s based on Zen Buddhism and has come into our mainstream culture, even in more conservative groups. I recently listened to the podcast of the US Surgeon General with his friend Jon Kabat Zin, who made mindfulness mainstream. His system "Mindfulness-Based Stress Reduction" (MBSR) has been used in prisons, hospitals, schools and the military.

I confess to once saying, "I haven't got time to sit cross-legged on a mat and I'd really rather not hear what's going on inside my head, thank you." Perhaps you currently think this. But as the saying goes, the less time you have, the more you should do it.

I was formerly not very good at sitting still unless I was completely exhausted. However, I have come to really value this practice as part of my day. And who amongst us wouldn't want to take a little time out when it has so many benefits? Sitting down and taking a beat has benefits out of all proportion to the time it takes out of your day.

A large number of studies have confirmed many benefits, including these below.

In all populations from college students to marines, it undoubtedly reduces the stress response. Studies have confirmed that regular mindfulness practice both reduces stress and improves wellbeing and even has an anti-aging effect. It increases telomerase, an enzyme responsible for the maintenance of the length of telomeres – those little DNA protein structures that, if healthy, hold the key to delaying or even reversing cellular ageing. So, no-effort anti-aging, which saves a fortune on the lotions and potions that promise we will all soon look like those twenty-year-old lovelies in the advertisements.

It also reinforces positive emotions, enhances engagement and builds resilience. Not a bad return for taking a moment or several out of your busy day. Also, and this is a really good thing research tells us, it does not have to be repeated a lot to have a really positive effect on your stress response.

(N.B. If you are or think you may be chronically depressed or have suffered trauma, you should discuss the use of mindfulness with a doctor/therapist who is looking after you.)

There are many ways to incorporate mindfulness into your day. How you find time for it is up to you. The optimal time is fifteen to twenty minutes but you can start with five. As with most things, consistency is the key. If you can do five minutes reasonably regularly, please do. Maybe bring it into your morning quiet time or perhaps you can bookend the end of a working day. If you use a car for work, taking five minutes before getting out and going into the house can be self-care for you and for the people who live in your house!

Try Dr Benson's (of the Benson Henry Institute at Harvard) 'Relaxation Response' for five minutes.

Here's how you do it. I've produced an audio for you to follow along[3], but you could also take these instructions and set a timer on your phone with one of the calmer ringtones. You can set a timer for a minimum of five minutes or more if you like.

You need two things: a bit of quiet and a word (a positive one, please!) or a sound, number or phrase that you can repeat.

Other thoughts will inevitably come to mind and when they do Dr Benson recommends saying, *oh, well*. Don't worry if you say *oh, well* quite a lot at first. It is perfectly normal and the *oh, wells* will dial down as you practise.

First, sit comfortably, then relax the muscles in your feet, your calves, your thighs and all the way up through your body. Gently roll your head/neck to release the tension.

Then breathe slowly, if you can, and with each out breath say the number, word or phrase.

If the thoughts come up, say *oh, well* and return to the breath and to saying your word or number.

Keep that going until the end of the session.

When the timer sounds, keep your eyes closed and let the day-to-day thoughts come back in. Slowly open your eyes and take a moment before you get up and start your day. You may feel slightly dizzy if you get up too quickly, which is normal, but just take it gently and see how you feel.

CREATE TIME

You can benefit from creating even a minute of time to take a time-out. A single minute out of your day somewhere where you won't be disturbed to break up your activity is not too much to do for yourself. Sit down, close your eyes, shut down as many tabs as possible, and do nothing for just a minute. Time it if you want to. Without fail, my clients all say that minute feels really long at first, so start with that. It will build and these short little oases of time which sometimes occur in times and places that are not obvious can help you through the busiest of days.

It is put beautifully by Jon Kabat Zin:

> "Just this moment,
> Just this breath,
> Just this sitting here,
> Just this being human,
> Just this. Just this."

4

RELATIONSHIPS

"When we love we always strive to become better than we are. When we strive to become better than we are everything around us becomes better too."

— PAULO COELHO

Although this is the third of the Permah pillars, relationships is arguably the most fundamental pillar of our wellbeing and happiness. "No man is an island," wrote John Donne, even though when things are not going as well as they should in this aspect of our lives, we sometimes wish that we could go and live on one.

When talking about relationships, I mean not only those we have with our loved ones, our family, and our friends but also those we have at work and in the wider community. The largest study ever of human behaviour at Harvard, which deals with longevity, indicates that the best sign of longevity and happiness is that of strong social connections.

BELONGING THEORY

"Other people matter."

— DR CHRISTOPHER PETERSON

There is now a science of belonging. So, what do we know and why is it useful?

Researchers have discovered that happiness is not a solo project. "It is scientifically correct to say that no one reaches their full potential in isolation."[1] Further studies of longevity of the population in so-called blue zone countries across continents from Sardinia to Okinawa have shown that a characteristic of longevity is that their residents put family first and keep socially engaged. The right types of relationships keep you young, which is a good reason to get good at them.

One of my closest friends, Pen, is twenty years older than me and yet there has never seemed to be a divide. I think many of us have experienced a friendship like this in our lives. I met her when I was a young barrister in my early twenties and she was a well-respected solicitor. In my eyes and the eyes of my contemporaries, she was a real role model who was really good at what she did but was cool and fun too. Her home was always a hub for a variety of interesting people. Her sons and her sons' friends, were lodgers there from time to time, and I was too. She is so interested in people and ideas and her house was a great place to be. She's always been with me throughout my career as a great sounding board, as I have been to her also, I hope. As well as being a career role model, she gave me an insight into how we can keep ourselves engaged and vital. She retired only last year at seventy-five, still as engaged and interested as she ever was. This bears out the science that being with other people gives you another entry to positivity.

CAN'T BUY ME LOVE... OR GREAT RELATIONSHIPS

If having more and more money leads to hedonic adaptation (i.e., the more money we get the more money we need), the contrary is true of relationships. When you build your relationships, your discontent at not having enough disappears.

Here is a fabulous example of this working in practice: Luke worked at McDonalds in Cardiff. He met his soon-to-be wife there and got on really well with his coworkers and regular customers and really valued those relationships. Luke had a big win on the lottery and, as you may expect, gave up his job at McDonalds. He had the wedding and honeymoon of his dreams, bought a house and was living, as he put it, "his best life". Luke later featured in national newspapers – *not* as one of the lottery winners who blew his fortune and ended up in poverty but when he returned to his job at McDonalds because he *wanted* to. He explained that one year into his rich life, as happy as he was with his wife and family, he missed being at work. He loved being part of a team and missed the people and customers he worked with. His colleagues who had been delighted for his success welcomed him back. The only difference the lottery made to him was that now he gets a taxi to work on the odd occasion he doesn't want to walk. Other people really do matter…

In our fast-paced world, it may be useful to slow down and to really understand why good relationships matter for us and, sometimes more importantly, for the people around us. There's a strong self-interest in knowing this, because again, for very little effort, we can gain so much. Generally, we want to get along with people and we have a very basic instinct to help others. Here is some of the why and the how to improve relationships.

People with good relationships have higher levels of self-esteem, greater life satisfaction, faster recovery from illness or disease, and lower stress. Studies have shown that having supportive social ties adds nine years of healthy life.

We have seen recently that social attachments improve in times of crisis. When we experience adverse circumstances, it is in our natures to come together. During Covid in the UK we expressed our support for workers in the NHS. Yes, of course they needed financial support and better care, yet people were happy to get onto their doorsteps and show support and gratitude. This may have been at a time when they did not know their neighbours, but new associations were formed. Many noticed that when we all stayed in, the levels of community that our grandparents enjoyed came back for a time and there was an awareness of the sense of community that we had lost.

Belonging theory reflects the desire of humans to belong. That desire and the associated fear of being isolated leads to a reluctance to break social bonds and relationships, sometimes very much to the person's detriment. Scientifically speaking, we are at least as reluctant to break bonds as we are to create new ones.

Another feature of belonging theory is that our intimate relationships shape our thinking. People generally think a lot more about their relationships than they do other parts of their lives. My 'law girls' and I used to joke back in the day that if we put as much effort into our careers as we did our latest romantic dilemmas, we'd have been the Lady Chief Justice by now (senior judge in England and Wales). It is interesting that we process information about our close partners differently.

The theory of belonging demonstrates that when we are intertwined with connection, we are said to feel other people's emotions. It is said that we strive to make people happy because we don't want to experience their pain. We want them to be happy because *we* want to be happy. Social pain triggers the same response in the brain as physical pain. It is true that you can really be heartbroken.

We have to be aware that we are so tuned in to connection and belonging, that we can interpret even the most minimal of social cues as rejection. Our minds take over and we construct complete scenarios for why X must have happened or why Y behaved in this way, and we work from a negative bias. I think experience tells us that it's not always about us, but we are battling the way that we are wired.

RELATIONSHIPS, FAMILY AND TRYING TO KEEP ALL THE PLATES SPINNING

One of the issues I frequently encounter with people who are working very hard is that they tend to default to keeping up with work and just coping with the basics of everything else, hoping that it will all be fine. The background of my profession taught me that the work day extends into the evening, at least a day on the weekend and sometimes two. Many of those I work with as clients in different professions have the same experience. Juggling work, the commute, spending a few hours with the children before they go to bed, and then starting work again leaves very little time for anything else, especially a partner. This is unsustainable in the long term and you may be able to see what or who is not getting the attention that they might. It is not that there is no connection but that there is no time for them individually or for the relationship, which in their quieter moments they (or you) fear for.

Many of us can be in relationships where we take it for granted that we are ok, or in a relationship that is put off until the kids go to school, or until they leave home… we may be storing up problems for ourselves simply because we just don't have the time.

THE LAZY GUIDE TOOLS TO KEEPING RELATIONSHIPS AT THE FOREFRONT

We can do small low-effort things to enhance someone else's experience. As you have chosen to be with them, I assume you quite like them and you would want to increase their happiness levels. As you may have gathered, doing that will also enhance yours.

These are a few little things that you can add into the day to reestablish that connection and increase the positive emotions quotient.

Be appreciative. Take a minute or two to tell them why you are grateful to them. Too often we know what we really like and admire about our person but don't ever say it. Perhaps it is the little things you notice they do. We all like to be appreciated. If we don't feel as though we are, our minds can play tricks on us and make up reasons why nothing is being said.

Be interested. Ask them what's going on in their day. Take some of that time you have squeezed out in the morning by not picking up your phone to find out how their day is going to go. In the evening, be interested in what has happened in their day. Everyone enjoys a good download. Here is a tip for you if you are a solution-focused person: unless you are asked, this is not a time for you to come up with a solution. Just listen and be interested.

Do something – anything – together. Do something one of you likes doing. Take turns and time out to be in each other's worlds. On these mythical date nights (do try and get them) or during any time together, try to let it be a media-free zone. We've all seen couples at the table with their heads in their phones, off in another realm. Are they texting each other?

As well as these easy tools, there are other really good ways to enhance communication and appreciation within all kinds of relationships.

THE COSTS OF BEING A DOWNER

Science tells us that for every negative comment or criticism you make to someone close to you, you should say five compensatory positive things to rebalance it in the mind of the recipient. Faithful to this being a lazy guide, your takeaway here is to be less negative and critical in the first place!

FRIENDSHIPS ARE SOME OF OUR GREATEST RELATIONSHIPS

Three good friends are all you need to be happy, so the science says.

Friendships are really important to us and when they end it can have the same effect as a relationship breaking up, yet these are some of the relationships that tend to fall by the wayside as they go down our list of priorities. Bearing in mind that some of these people are your three o'clock in the morning red button friends, try to make space for them too. At the risk of sounding like a broken record, it is about awareness and using a tiny bit of time for intention.

We make time for all the things we'd rather not be doing so why not make it for the things we love? It may take a bit of effort, as our spontaneity goes when we get older, but it is worth it, and so are you, and so are they.

Some of the strategies for happy coupledom can be used for your friends. Some of you have friends who are closer than your partners in many ways.

You have friends who have been in your life for years. You grew up together but you really don't see them, just because life is too busy. Time with them holds great memories, though. When social media reminds you of such-and-such a memory or a significant date comes up in the calendar, perhaps do more than repost or like a memory. Actually, get in touch. It's a nice solution to your slight embarrassment for the inadvertent lack of contact.

COME TOGETHER *IN REAL LIFE*

This is so basic but we often forget. We can all come together in times of crisis but why don't we come together *just because?* I am close to my girl cousins but we only ever came together at funerals... so we arranged a weekend together. It took some doing but it was amazing.

Reactivate your mutual interests. I have recently started doing this as my best friend and I, who live in different cities, can't seem to get together to go out. Other things always take priority. However, we both love tennis. Lo and behold, apparently, we can make time to get together to play. We get time for a margarita and a catch up too – it hardly cements our former rock chick status, but we do what we can when we can.

And when you do get together – hugging. If you are not a hugger, trot past this one but hugging is highly recommended. The last few socially-distanced years when hugs, handshakes or even a reassuring pat on the shoulder or touch on the arm were not allowed showed us how appropriate contact is such a part of our day-to-day lives. We all need (consensual) human touch so go on… hug away.

Create new routines or rituals for you and your friends and really dial that in. You used to have your places where you hung out so find new ones; take it in turns to book a dinner in different types of restaurants; challenge each other to do something you've never done: it needn't be extreme sports, just something new.

And what should you do when you really haven't got time? Even small efforts can make a vast difference. Check in regularly with others, offering to help if you can. Send an actual handwritten note or card. Receiving something thoughtful can lift someone's day and if it is a random gesture, it makes it all the more impactful. Set aside time for calls when you know you both have time. A client of mine whose best friend lives away and works really difficult shift patterns has worked out a time for a weekly call when they are both free and awake enough to enjoy the conversation.

In all types of relationships, there are those who drain you rather than energise you. (A word of caution: we can all behave in this way as well, especially if we are caught up in what is happening to us.) There are some friends you feel depleted by. Sometimes it's difficult when they have been in your life for a long time. We all have our bad times and being loyal to your friends through those is of course the right thing to do. But what of those who don't seem to think that you have other things that you need to attend to? Those who relentlessly bombard you with their problems and seem oblivious to yours? You might usefully ask this question: if you met them today, would you become friends with them?

Think carefully about how you might withdraw from those relationships: their dramas can't become your distraction. It's no good for you and no good for them. We all want to help and we all want to do our best, but there is a time to draw a line for yourself. You're spreading yourself too thin already.

IMPROVE YOUR COMMUNICATION WITH THE LOVE OF YOUR LIFE, YOUR FAMILY AND ALMOST EVERYONE WHO MATTERS

This exercise is called *active constructive listening*. It is a brilliant way to become closer to anyone who matters in your life.

When this formed part of the US Army study (Chapter 2) the feedback was extremely positive. When the participants were reporting on using this exercise in family life, they were appreciative of the depth it added to their relationships. Sadly, comments such as, "If I knew this then I don't think I'd be divorced now / would be closer to my kids," were not unusual. They also noted a change in their attitude to junior ranks' performance. Their questions no longer came from the negative which allowed them to properly support their soldiers' achievements and understand reasons for perceived failure.

The work on active constructive listening by Shelley Gable, Professor of Psychology, and colleagues at the University of California has shown that how you celebrate with someone is more predictive of positive relationships than how you disagree. So how does it work?

This is really a way to enhance your communication with loved ones or colleagues. It requires only a little tweak to what I suspect most of you do already.

The exercise is called *active constructive responding*. There are four ways of responding:

Active constructive
Passive constructive
Active destructive
Passive destructive

Let's take an example scenario.

Someone announces on returning home to their partner that they had got a promotion.

A passive constructive response could be: *Oh, that's great! Well done! I'm having a glass of wine; do you want one?* (All said with no expression.)

An active destructive response: *Did you? Ok, but won't that mean you're spending more time at the office and travelling more? You know how you hate packing.* (All said with a slight frown.)

A passive destructive response: ignores what they've just been told

.... You didn't bring the shopping: there's nothing in the cupboard. What are we going to do for food? (Nonverbal cues are little or no eye contact and turning away.)

The **active constructive** response is to say: *Congratulations! Really well done! Let's open that good bottle of wine we were saving to celebrate... so tell me how were you told. Were you called into the boss's office? Did you guess what she was about to say? What did she actually say? That must have made you feel...* (Nonverbal cues are eye contact, genuine smiles, a hug or touching.)

You can see the difference. When you give an active constructive response, you reinforce the positive by asking for more details. Only one or two questions about what happened amplifies the experience for the person who is receiving it. It will make them happy and if done genuinely it will make you happy too. This interaction will have a positive spiral and your person, teen or colleague will be open to sharing more of their experiences with you. As they let you more into their day-to-day, you'll feel better about it too and as you do, you become more adept at using this valuable skill. It really is a double win and takes only a little thought.

WHAT LOVE LANGUAGE DO YOU SPEAK?

Find out at what is your love language quiz:

www.5lovelanguages.com[2]

This interesting quiz can be done by you and your partner, more grown-up kiddos and friends.

We all experience things in different ways and how we feel appreciated is one of those differences. This quiz tells you what your 'love language®' is. Do try it and see. This helps us understand why sometimes we don't feel appreciated or even why we don't feel loved, though the person we are with is demonstrating what he or she thinks is love.

Perhaps when you get your results and compare them with your partner's you will see where the disconnect has arisen. You may feel underappreciated despite all your partner does for you, even though they are expressing their love in the way they know how. Understanding how we experience love is the key to understanding each other. It is also a really good indicator as to how to deal with your teen.

AND FINALLY... GRATITUDE

Yes, gratitude is here again, because being in gratitude makes you feel better. On my first foray into the new world of self-development, I was asked to write a gratitude letter in the context of relationships. I wrote it to my mum and posted it to her. I had a lot to be grateful for to both her and my dad. I didn't get a chance to say this to him so I wrote to her. I told her what she meant to me and how she and Dad had given me the best possible start and support. They had always said they didn't mind what I did as long as it made me happy (and clearly as long as it wasn't criminal). With that kind of loving, supportive background I had the space to do what I chose and be who I chose. I thanked her for giving me the love of reading and writing. I could read a way before I went to school and she opened my mind to a vast world of possibility in storytelling. She wasn't ill, and there was no acute problem in her life that she needed cheering up about – I just sent it and I am glad that I did. It meant so much to her and to me. I found it in her dresser after she had died.

The letter doesn't have to be grand: it can be a simple acknowledgement or a card just to say thank you. Do it, because it's easy and it feels good.

5

MEANING AND PURPOSE – WHY MEANING MATTERS AND WHY WE ALL NEED TO MATTER

"Success, like happiness, cannot be pursued. It must ensue as the unintended side effect of one's personal dedication to a cause greater than one's self."

— MIHALY CSIKZENTMIHALYI

This sounds quite a grand topic and actually, it is. Meaning in our lives is based on feelings of significance and mattering. It is about being able to make sense of life and have a purpose. Meaning and purpose is an antidote to experiencing life as a sometimes-exhausting treadmill. It answers for us the often-asked question *what is this all about?* Knowing your life has meaning and understanding your purpose can reframe your life and keep you going when things get really tough.

You can see where you are in relation to this by taking the *meaning in life* questionnaire. The meaning in life questionnaire is the work of Dr Michael Steger and he provides this valuable resource. His website is: www.michaelfsteger.com

Again, awareness is key. Before we go on to discuss how you can understand how to amplify meaning and purpose in your life with little effort, a little background may help.

WHY US MATTERING MATTERS

Traditionally, the way we behave was thought to be dictated by the two major drivers of pleasure and pain, that is, the pursuit of pleasure and the avoidance of pain. While that is true – who wouldn't want to avoid pain and have pleasurable life experiences? – there has been a piece missing.

Why do people who seemingly have everything – talent, career success and apparently great relationships – feel so empty? We live in a society that reinforces the concept of *I will be happy when... I get x job... when I make x amount of cash... when I find a great relationship...* and so on. Yet when we achieve what we think will make us happy, there's still a nagging or empty feeling telling us there must be something more.

So why aren't we happy? We know happiness does not come from things. It is not money and past a certain point, it may not even be health. A study of those who became paraplegic and those who became lottery winners showed that after one year their happiness levels had returned to baseline.

We need meaning in our lives. It doesn't matter where you are from or what you do, you can attach meaning to any situation or task. The janitor study is an example – you can be the most renowned surgeon in your field but if you value your job only for the material benefits it brings, your level of happiness will be lower than the hospital janitor who thinks his role is to make things as pleasant as he possibly can for people.

HOW DOES MEANING SHOW UP IN OUR LIVES?

It is a basic human need to feel that our lives have meaning. It is the sort of thing that gets you out of bed every morning. *But wait,* you say… *I have to get up every morning and go to work or someone will come and take away the furniture.* I understand that. However, except for those with a private income, we have to spend large parts of our day working so it makes sense to analyse how we can best expend our energies while we are there and to gain as much benefit as we can.

Let's start from the basis that meaning is actually a basic human need, not a nice to have. When we don't have it, we feel empty, listless and valueless. Having meaning is the key to feeling that life is worth living. It helps you keep going when it feels like you are swimming against the tide. It leads to optimism that can help you through the most stressful times. Life is better and you are contented. Also, as a by-product of expanding meaning, you become more productive at work which can't be a bad thing.

What creates a meaningful life? Research has shown that there are four pillars that support a life full of meaning:

Belonging
Purpose
Storytelling
Transcendence

Knowing what they are enables us to expand into them. As ever, there are low-effort ways for you to implement some of these things and bring your life so much benefit.

THE LAZY GUIDE TOOLS TO ADD MEANING TO YOUR LIVES

Belonging. All of us have a need to be respected and valued. We want to pay attention to others and have that returned. There is a need to feel you are not alone. The connections you have are important to you. We can create meaning from this need to belong and enhance our own and others' experiences.

Find your tribe. Outside of your family, you can find tribe groups that you can belong to online or (preferably) in real life. Get together with people who have a favourite team, politics, causes or interests in common. Commonality is a way to feel you really belong.

We have become more isolated within society. We know that younger people are expressing loneliness as a problem. Friendships are precious but we struggle to keep friendships up in our day-to-day lives. We are losing spoken communication. I've noticed that outside of a close circle of friends, the etiquette is to voice note and message. Our 'IRL' experiences are narrow.

Simply asking, "Can I help?" is a good way to start. Offering help to a friend or colleague in any small way you can contribute is gold for them to hear and it can make you feel good too.

Volunteering. Even a small amount of time spent volunteering makes a difference. Most of us are naturally inclined to want to help if we can, which you can see in the donations made in the wake of disasters in other countries, even in times of recession. Not that you personally need one but there is a selfish reason for being altruistic: it makes us feel really good. A Harvard Business School study of happiness in 136 countries found that people who made generous charitable donations appropriate to their means are the happiest of all the populations. The 1980's saw the discovery of the 'helper's high' which has been confirmed by numerous studies. Pleasure centres in the brain light up and you have the same feelings when you are the giver as the recipient experiences. It increases your feelings of self-worth, you feel stronger and more in control, calmer and less prone to depression – what is not to like?

Mentoring. Another excellent way to contribute is by mentoring either in your community or at work. It is your chance to give back. I know you are busy but some of the busiest people I know take the time to mentor and volunteer. Identify your strengths and find a mentoring role that uses them. Being a role model reinforces your purpose and the people you mentor will see and receive positive examples. The ripple effect just keeps spreading...

A little can go a very long way. You don't have to make huge donations. Don't underestimate the power of a smile and a hello to someone you see who might need it – it can at the very least raise someone's day and it could actually save a life.

In his work on suicide, Robert Holden[1] describes how one man who attempted suicide on the Golden Gate Bridge left a note in his apartment which read, *if one person smiles at me, I will not jump off the bridge.* Tragically, no one did and the man jumped. Amazingly he survived the fall and was able to be saved by clinging on to a sealion! He became an advocate for suicide prevention and tells his story in order to help others. Afterwards, he was asked if a smile would have saved him from jumping, and he said yes it would. This is not an uncommon response. The motif of suicide prevention month has been designed as a genuine smile. You may not be able to save a life but you can make someone else's quality of life better by doing such a simple thing.

WHAT ABOUT WORK?

When you feel that there is personal growth as well as professional growth, when you have a shared sense of purpose, and when you find meaning in service of other people, these are indicators that your work has meaning for you. This can be difficult to see when you are overwhelmed and the concept of work/life balance seems a distant memory.

It is optimum if your work reflects your values and your talents and if you are aligned with the purpose of the company or organisation where you spend your working life. If not, in the current climate, finding a role or company in which you can use those might seem a luxury, but in the meantime, there is no harm in thinking about and getting clear on what that could look like.

If your job is just that – a job – you can find meaning within it by using your talents and strengths and paying attention to how you can add them to the day-to-day tasks.

It is often the people we work with who buoy us up when things get too overwhelming. We are adjusting to getting back into the workspaces and while working from home can sometimes be a blessing, seeing (most) of our colleagues at work and interacting with them can add something pleasant to the grind. In these days of more and more remote events, you could think about spending some more 'IRL' time such as coffee dates, or informal walking meetings if you can manage them, and generally being actively interested in what they are all about.

DON'T FORGET THE GOOD YOU DO TOO!

When you are dealing with crises and deadlines, you lose track of yourself and what you do well. Add more meaning to your work life by compiling an audit of what you have achieved – and really appreciate it. We tend to miss this out, but it can enhance our sense of personal growth. I always have encouraged trainees to address this and now I encourage my coachees to do the same. Start small and examine what has gone well on a day-to-day basis in order to focus on the positive.

PURPOSE – LIFE IS HAPPIER WHEN YOU KNOW YOUR WHY

Whether you have a purpose in life or you don't, I'm not here to tell you that you must have one or what that purpose should be. I'm here to explain how life, particularly when it gets choppy, is a whole lot easier to deal with if you have one… or, interestingly, if you are *looking for one*. A purpose is a fundamental means of grounding yourself when the ground around you is moving. So, what is a 'why' and how (if you want to) do you get one?

PURPOSE AT HOME

Your purpose can be your family. An experience in my own family totally reinforced this for me. Please be assured there is a happy ending. My father had a heart attack in his early forties and was clinically dead for a period. Happily, he was resuscitated; having a consultant called Dr Lazarus (I'm not joking) looking after him may have helped.

Years later he talked to me about it. He said that the feeling was one of being overwhelmingly tired in a way he'd never experienced before. He said it felt like it would be the easiest thing to let go but he had a strong sense of wanting to be with us – mum, my brother and me – and that stopped him giving in to the tiredness. Personally, I also think he was desperate not to miss out on something as he was, to put it mildly, curious about life! But his strong value of looking after people kept driving him on.

We were told he wouldn't make it through the night, yet he lived until he was eighty. He was the epitome of resilience and lived by his motto that life isn't a rehearsal: you have to make it count.

PURPOSE AT WORK

Having a sense of purpose is that thing that gets you out of bed in the morning. It is the feeling that something you do makes a difference. The purpose need not be noble or grand and you don't have to be a surgeon being flown out to perform lifesaving surgery or an athlete representing your country. (I am writing this as England's Lionesses have reached the World Cup final.)

You may think that meaning or a calling is only available to a select few, but in a 2018 study Seligman et al surveyed two thousand full-time employees within the income bracket of $40,000 dollars to $200,000 across all age ranges and genders. The result was that almost everyone wanted their employment to be more of a calling than a job. When asked how meaningful their current roles were, people gave their jobs a meaning quotient of 49 percent.

This, however, is the shocker: on average, people were willing to sacrifice a huge 23 percent of their future earnings to always have a job that would be highly meaningful. We must balance that against the fact that in 2018 people spent an average of 17.5 percent of their income on a mortgage. They were willing to put more meaningful employment before a house. Things have changed much in the world since then, but it really does demonstrate how much we want meaning in our work and want to feel that what we do matters.

Understanding the types of approaches to work may help explain where we are on the scale and how to elevate it if we want to.[2] It also helps demonstrate that the important thing is not what you do but what you *think* about what you do. Whatever you do can make a difference for people every day.

There are three types of approaches to work:

Job approach – focused on financial rewards and necessity. The job is a means to an end, to allow you to enjoy life out of work. You move on for better pay.

Career approach – focused on professional advancement. You take pride in accomplishment, promotion, and social standing. You leave when the promotions stop.

Calling – focused on fulfilling work. You keep at it no matter what because you feel it is socially valuable work.

All of these are valid and if you are comfortable where you are that's great, but if things start to become a little hollow or if you feel that when you've got to the top of your particular tree you'll want something more (and many people do), you can dial down and look at what your purpose is in life.

The great thing about purpose is that looking for it can have all the benefits of actually having it. Also, your purpose can change as you go on in life.

DON'T OVERDO IT AND DON'T BE A MARTYR TO THE CAUSE

Career (and to an extent *calling*), particularly when it aligns with being in your tribe, can have a downside of which you should be aware. It can take over your whole life to the detriment of successful relationships and positive emotions. This has come up for a lot of the people with whom I work.

I know in my profession, and perhaps you may be familiar with this, that the amount of time I have to put into the work both in the day and the evening puts other aspects of my life in difficulty if I don't manage it. You may need to guard against freezing people out. Sometimes a calling is indistinguishable from workaholism in that it has the same negative effects. For those who may be afflicted, a way to approach this is to 'eat some pie'! Imagine your week as a pie: how big a slice is work? Are you overeating? Would a smaller slice serve you better, what could change to make things a little more palatable for everyone including you?[3]

REALLY SET BOUNDARIES

Decide how many hours a task needs and give it just that. Don't be the person who is always on call or who always covers. Going at full tilt all the time is not good for you or the people you want to help. Maybe you have this tendency or, if not, you will know someone who does. Being ill through overwork does not serve you or the people that you want to serve. This applies not only to work but to familial obligations: it's no good you getting ill when all the family needs propping up.

FIND YOUR PURPOSE AND GET BACK ON TRACK

I have experienced what I think is one of the most influential examples of change work. I would love to guide you through it 'IRL' however you can experience this eyes-closed process in the comfort of your own home.[4] It is not hypnotherapy, to reassure those who do not want to experience that but it is nonetheless powerful.

It is called neuro-levels, the work of Robert Diltz, and is similar to Maslow's hierarchy of needs but goes deeper. Do try it because can't hurt and it may well help a lot.

STORYTELLING

We all want to feel like we matter and storytelling is a way of achieving this: it is said that "Mattering is the story we tell ourselves to explain our own existence." Telling your story of why you matter gives your wellbeing a tremendous boost.

Its opposite is feeling empty, feeling that nothing we do matters and therefore we question why we do it. We give up because we feel we don't matter and don't make a difference.

We love stories. Hearing the stories of those of us who have gone before us, especially what they did and achieved, can help us make sense of the world. We love stories of growth and we are inspired by people who have overcome unbelievable odds and circumstances to thrive.

The stories we tell ourselves about ourselves define our world. As with all stories, they get stronger and added to in the retelling, which is good if they are positive, not so good, if they are not. But the good news is that we are the authors and we can always look at whatever has happened to us in our lives through a different lens. For some it may mean through the lens of therapy; for others it may mean simply reflecting on what else past events could mean.

Outside hugely traumatic experiences, it is useful to see what you have done in the past and utilise it now. You can review things in the light of learning or growth. A growth mindset here helps enormously: this is the ability to see things you consider failures as learning opportunities.

When you tell a story about yourself and about your life, listen out for the language that you use. Perhaps you will hear *I'm always... it's always like this... I never...* or *I'm too old...* If you tell yourself these things, that is where you stay. What you do matters and who you are matters so be careful of the negative stories you tell yourself. Words have power.

Our minds are very easily influenced towards the negative. Approaching what's happened with an open mind and one that is willing to learn provides us with a new and positive story.

You can think about a negative event and pick it apart to see if something good came out of it. You can tell yourself a story about how you don't belong or have imposter syndrome or you can use that feeling to assess the reality of the situation. Sometimes it's just that you're new somewhere, that's all. Maybe you are somewhere you have always wanted to be, surrounded by people who are ahead of you or whom you admire. We all have something to contribute and having energy and enthusiasm for where you are brings something to the people around you too. I see it a lot in work with bright, enthusiastic pupils and juniors generating affectionate smiles from case-hardened 'veterans".

Making 'the mess your message' is at the heart of purpose and resilience. Taking an event that has disturbed you or even one that was hugely traumatic and rewriting your story can become your life's work, as we saw in the story of the suicide survivor. We all know of famous examples but I'm inspired by the people with whom I've come into contact over the years who have used the worst that could happen to a person to become shining lights for those they can help. It is in the telling of those stories again and again that people find hope.

Another way to look at your story is from a legacy point of view – how would you like to be remembered and what would you want people to say about you? It is often said that people at the end of their lives don't recount their successes in the office. They talk about the people who have touched their lives and how the world has been made slightly better for their having been here. This point of view is not for everyone but it'll help you focus on what your meaning is. If you have the time, why not?

Here's mine: a good daughter, sister, partner, friend, someone who wanted to learn as much as she could about life and how it works, a good helper who wanted people to be happy, and she made a few more people happy than she irritated with her constant questions. And oh, yes, she contributed to... world peace!

TRANSCENDENCE

Here is where my more cynical friends perhaps start to feel a little resistance... She's going to start talking about meditation and we told you we haven't got time or worse, she'll be asking us to align with a higher power. So, for you, my friends, before I unashamedly do both, here's an incentive and a bit of neuroscience to ease your path. However, it is for the rest of you, too, as we all need a bit of reinforcement.

Dr Lisa Miller[5] and a team at Yale conducted a series of MRIs on volunteers who were asked to think about a spiritual experience. Her results revealed an area of the brain she described as "a natural docking station for spiritual awareness." There are two parts of the brain wired to accept the spiritual. We are naturally preprogrammed to be in awe!

WHAT IS TRANSCENDENCE AND HOW DO WE GET IT IN OUR LIVES?

Transcendence is a state in which everything – the noise of everyday life and its problems – fades away. The obvious place is of course within organised religion. Many of us only resort to prayer when things go badly wrong and we bargain with or make promises to the higher power. Some of my military friends have described becoming deeply religious at certain points in their tours. While that may not be for you, it seems that across all divides we are looking for something 'more', something greater than us.

Transcendence is not only to be found in quiet churches or soaring cathedrals. It may be there are other cathedrals of sorts. I would suggest you can have a deeply spiritual experience standing on the terraces at the National Stadium in Wales as part of the crowd singing the national anthem. Exposure to art or music in all its forms and whichever way you enjoy it can take you to a completely different place and uplift you out of the ordinary.

GET OUT IN NATURE

The awe centres in our brains are clearly activated by nature, which is why so many of us stop and watch a sunset. I see it here on the beach at New Year. There seems to be a compulsion to come and watch the sun go down on the year. Sure, the parties start later but it's generally quiet as people sit together and watch the sunset.

Time after time, when the 'awesome' has been studied the participants have been shown to become less self-centred than before and behave in a more generous fashion. You'll have noticed the experience seems to be enhanced when there are people there too.

So go to church, listen to great music, dance, meditate, go to the rugby or watch the sunset – these are all amazing experiences in their own right that take us out of the here and the now and give us a taste of the divine.

6

ACCOMPLISHMENT – BEING A GOAL-GETTER

"Success is a journey, not a destination. The doing is more important than the outcome."

— ARTHUR ASHE

WHY ARE GOALS IMPORTANT AND WHAT, INDEED, IS THE RUSH?

You may wish to know what's with the talk about goals, this being the lazy guide and all. I know that a lot of the time we are just trying to get by with a vague notion that the goal is to one day soon be lying under a palm tree with a cocktail in hand. That, I concede, is absolutely valid but there is something in us all that drives us to do more. There is a basic curiosity about what is around the corner and what we can do. When we don't have something to work towards, listlessness overtakes us and we lose focus and control.

WHY GOALS ARE GOOD

Having goals gives us a sense of purpose, and working towards goals bolsters our self-esteem; they add structure and meaning to our lives. This is why retirees often have difficulties adjusting and there are now initiatives to assist with retirement directed towards personal and emotional goals. Goals also often lead us to engaging with others. There is a strong element of involving other people and getting their assistance.

Goals help us master our time as we have larger goals and subgoals to work towards. This helps us divide our time. Who hasn't buckled under an always expanding to-do list where things never get crossed off?

Goals or taking steps towards them can keep us going in moments of crisis (although of course certain events are too catastrophic). I can personally attest to this. After having a particularly traumatic few months with bereavement, I was alone at the family home in Wales when Covid struck and lockdown happened. I managed to get Covid right in the period when we thought it was going to be for three weeks but turned into heaven knows how long. I was stuck so I had a goal of busting out of solitary with all my faculties intact (I joke, but it was rather a test of one's resilience). I reactivated what I had done in the past, which I knew was a baseline. I had a book with a list of things I was going to do every day and I ticked them off until we were allowed to travel and I could go home. This baseline actually provided the basis for the work I do now. So, I ticked off tasks every day and although I didn't feel my best, I was unreasonably pleased that I was doing it. I wrote down things I'd done that hadn't made the list so I could tick them off. I still have the book and the ticks today.

I know that what I was doing was setting smaller sub-goals every day. I took those supplements to get back to health. I did an online lunchtime meditation not only because it quietened my mind but because it was proven to increase confidence in what we have come to know as your response-ability.

We all have to live in the world and work either within the home or outside it. My argument is that it's helpful to know how to create a meaningful life by managing the way in which we do it. A key component of wellbeing is that we can look back on our lives with a sense of accomplishment. Steve Jobs said you can only join the dots when you look backwards. He cited intuition and following what for you is a meaningful path against perhaps the evidence around you at the time.

Looking at this pillar of positive psychology and that of meaning perhaps puts you in the best place to have the dots land in the right place in the here and now.

We will look at how you define success, and how you deal with setbacks and I will offer a suggestion or two on how to tweak your mindset. You could consider working towards goals as something which allows you to build up hope for the future. You can look back at what has and hasn't worked in the past but also really tap into what you have achieved in the past and how you achieved it, which will increase confidence about the future. By understanding where you came from, you can build towards that future.

So, what do you need to get there? Let's talk about willpower (or grit) and a growth mindset. This was all new to me once upon a time: I thought I hadn't got any willpower, and that grit was what you did with your teeth when people like me spoke about self-development. I had no idea what a growth mindset was as I was apparently a little bit fixed.

SELF-CONTROL AND WILLPOWER AND WHAT THE BUSY OR LAZY PERSON SHOULD KNOW

These are not everyone's strong points, for sure. Science aside, I do notice how I and others have a lot of willpower to do things we like but tend to fall away a little when we don't or when things get a little too hard.

So here are a few things I have learned about willpower from a number of studies I have read and (I must confess) a few TED talks I have watched.

You can think about willpower as a kind of self-control muscle. We exercise it to a greater or lesser extent every day. Some of us are more successful than others but if we try or are forced to try, we can still exercise it. Science tells us that we don't have a container of self-control for the day that is all gone when we've used it up and then we have to wait until the next day. Self-control is actually available to you when you are depleted, which is common sense if you think about it. If someone put a gun to your head, your motivation and willpower would skyrocket even if you were depleted. You can still use it if you have a good enough reason.

You can exercise this self-control muscle by, of all things, meditation!

You can expand your capacity by doing things a little differently. For example, if you are right-handed, you could use your left hand for drinking (not pints) or opening doors and so on. Start small because competence builds confidence.

Another really good way to harness self-control is to avoid putting yourself in situations where you are going to have to use your self-control. For example, you might say no to doing just one more case when you have a publication deadline to work towards!

You can be proactive by narrowing down the number of decisions that you have to make. We all know by now of Obama's grey suit, Mark Zuckerberg's grey t-shirts. By cutting down the decisions we have to make in a day - even the smallest ones - we increase our capacity for self-control. When we use social media, we unwittingly make hundreds of tiny decisions every day by deciding what we like and don't like, by replying to a comment, by judging an opinion – this all takes away from our limited energy resources for the day.

THE BEST TIME TO APPLY FOR PAROLE ON THE OFF CHANCE YOU NEED TO... OR, HOW TIMING CAN AFFECT OUR DECISION-MAKING ABILITY.

Decision-making and control is a function of parts of the brain that are fuelled with glucose.

A study[1] looked at the decisions of a Parole Board over a period of time. The judges there made between fourteen and thirty-five judgements a day. They had breaks for a snack at 10.30 and lunch at one. As the day went on there was an ever-decreasing grant of parole with the exception for hearings just after the snack break and lunch when positive results increased. Under twenty percent got parole after lunch, unless the hearing was right after lunch. This may be worth bearing in mind if you want to ask for something important at work or to bear in mind in your own day!

HOW DO YOU KNOW IF YOUR WILLPOWER/SELF-CONTROL IS DEPLETED?

Sometimes you might feel 'off', or rather, you might feel things more strongly. If you feel like this it might be a time to remind yourself that although you do have a lot of response-ability left, it would be optimum to restore and recover. Sometimes it is just good to shut the day down if you have something that really needs thought.

If you have to work or do anything in the evening, it could be better to just get things down if its written work and then shut the device. Come back to it in the morning when you're fresh.

THE FUTURE IS BRIGHTER AND YOUR FAILURES ARE LIGHTER WHEN YOU ADOPT A GROWTH MINDSET

Growth mindset is giving things a go, failing well and improving.

When you adopt a growth mindset you feel happier, less discouraged by difficulty, more resilient and don't tend to fall prey to comparisonitis. A fixed mindset avoids challenges as failure destroys it.

So many of us come from a fixed mindset. It is one that may not be as common now in education, I hope, but it seemed to be that whatever you were labelled, stuck. If you were praised for being clever maybe you linked that so closely with your identity that you were so scared to fail, and you either worked yourselves ridiculously hard or didn't try at all. It was better to give up than be found out by trying and failing.

People who are naturally talented at things do tend to fall prey to this labelling. This is not to say that some of them haven't worked hard to get where they are. As a population, we almost want people to have those talents to explain how they got there. There is a culture of calling people lucky when it's really all about hard work – for some reason we find others being lucky easier to deal with. However, we are all inspired by people who have come through the worst of times.

When I was younger, I heard someone say, "If I can't do something the first time then I don't do it." I'm very much afraid that might have been me.

The difference between growth and fixed mindsets can be encapsulated in the sentence: "This is all I can do rather than who knows what I can do." What you need is the belief that you can improve.

Failing well might be another way of looking at it. Edison said about his invention of the light bulb, "I haven't failed. I've just found ten thousand ways that won't work."

How do we get used to failure? If you fall off the horse you get back on, but do take a pause and see it as a learning opportunity.

Another good way of dealing with this is to have a bit of self-compassion. "If being hard on ourselves worked it would have worked by now." [2] We are all so relentlessly hard on ourselves – really try to silence that inner critic and also get some perspective. Speak to yourself as you would a friend in the same situation.

An often-used technique is to give the inner critic a name… someone from the past such as a teacher or a faux friend, or a boss, maybe. When the voice challenges you, tell it what you would if it were coming directly from them. I think you may be a little more inspired that way.

Do something – anything – that is a tiny step forward for you. By taking these small steps forward you change the way you feel about things.

A word about our children and the way we praise them, tapping into what we dealt with earlier. Praising a child for being clever may certainly be correct and raise their self-esteem in the short term, but we have seen the pressure that can put on the best of us. Praising a child for how they got there is perhaps the best way to deal with it so you praise through the verb rather than the adjective. When things do not go quite to plan, those children who are allowed to develop a fixed mindset may blame external forces. They might say, "It's the way they are marking this year," or, "That teacher's never liked me." Again, a better way to approach that is to acknowledge the work, if that's what they did, but maybe gently point out some learning opportunities. Better still, get them to think out loud about what they did *not* do – not from the voice of the critic but from the generally interested person to see how things can go on. Do your best but remember your best is not set in stone.

Goals are more about the lead-up to the realisation of the goal than the goal itself. It is the journey that gives us the dopamine. This is why, shortly after we reach our goals after a huge effort, we get the empty feeling of *what now? what next?* We often see it in sportsmen and women.

It may be that positive psychology can explain. There are *types* of goals: external extrinsic goals, goals that other people or society think we should aspire to, or intrinsic goals which are meaningful to us. Working toward goals that are meaningful and important to you is more satisfying than those that are chosen for you. Extrinsic goals are what society tells us we want, which usually involve money and status. They are valid sometimes because we have to be there or the mortgage or rent doesn't get paid. Sometimes you must grit through the unappealing side of work to get to a position that you do want. Intrinsic goals are personal to us and have meaning. They are fulfilling and give us a sense of autonomy, competence and relatedness which are some of our needs above the baseline of survival. Meaningful goals mean a meaningful and happy life.

HOPE THEORY

The appropriately named hope theory[3] helps us here. The aim is to put us in a positive and motivational state and our thought process is at the crux of that. It helps us think in a goal-oriented way and use pathways, finding different ways to reach the goals. It helps develop agency thinking which involves building confidence that you can make the change

Hope theory can be broken down into simple steps you can take to improve your life. I've got those steps for you here just in case you fancy getting off the sofa and springing into life... because as my dear pop would say, you're only here once, kiddo, so why not make it count?

"The Hope Map"

To begin, do the following:

Conceptualise or form the idea of your goals.
Brainstorm the strategies to get there.
State and maintain the motivation to get there.
Tap into the *why*.
Finally, get clear on who your support systems are and who are you going to need.

A little visualisation may help?

Remember a time when you achieved your goal. What did you do to get there? What small steps did you need? Who did you recruit to help you?

When you had achieved your goal how did you feel? Who was with you? What could you see and what could you hear?

There are end-state goals and process goals. End-state goals end when they have been achieved while process goals keep going through time. There are ways of approaching those goals. You can go for drastic change or gradual change, forming small, incremental habits that get you where you want to go. Or you could chunk down the goals.

Let's do this as an example through the goal of weight loss:

Choose a goal – drop a stone by X date.

Choose a repeated action – how you do it, for example, logging your food in an app.

Choose your approach – drastic action, chunking or gradual steps and then start taking action.

What will you do when you encounter blocks?
Who or what will you need to support you?

VISUALISATION

A powerful intervention which receives rave reviews is the *best possible self*-exercise. You can both imagine and write the best possible outcome for your future. Use the audio [4] and play it regularly on the path to achieving your goal. My former client, B, a junior surgeon, credits it with helping her through her fellowship.

It is said that our brains cannot distinguish between what is real and imagined and while that is not entirely true, we do know that visualisation is prevalent in elite sports.

The best possible self-visualisation is realistic and achievable, which engenders optimism. This, of course, is a proponent of hope. When you do the best future self-visualisation there has to be a level of realism. It is no good me imagining my best future self-winning Wimbledon. I'm clearly too old… Don't worry if that best future self is a little way from where you actually are. See a way ahead and make small steps towards that.

As Martin Seligman says, "The important thing about the imagination is that it gives you optimism". This exercise is one of the most recognised for boosting happiness. It does this by increasing hopefulness and focus specifically on what needs to change – it works as you are strengthening your optimism muscles thinking of the best rather than worst possible outcome.[5]

After you have completed the visualisation, take some time to make notes about it. What's not to love about imagining a successful future with some clear ways to get you there?

THE CONFIDENCE GAPS

Reluctance to pursue goals can be down to a number of things, including a desire to do nothing – no judgement here. But one of the biggest hurdles that some of us face is confidence. You don't have to have gone very far in any area of life to see that the people we admire have not always been confident or are not even as confident as they appear. Some people are naturally confident whether it is merited or not. But confidence does spring from competence and again I return to a theme. It is consistent effort, the consistent moving forward of the needle, which engenders genuine confidence. It's always good to ask people for help. From what can be a hard-bitten profession, one of the things I have always been able to do is ask for help. It is ok to say that you are new or that you have never done this before. As my pupil master used to say, when you think you know all there is to know, it's time for a radical rethink!

Confidence and consistency align really well with goal setting. When we set goals using the Hope Map, we tap into that learning from our past experiences. Knowing what our strengths are also helps.

Just take one aspect of confidence – public speaking. I have spent all my professional life speaking in public (with the added degree of difficulty of being dressed like I've come out of a Merchant Ivory film – wigs are hell for those of us with naturally curly hair – but I digress).

Over the years I've mentored our trainees (or pupils, as we still quaintly call them) and it is one of the better aspects of our profession that when we turn up to court and see the juniors foundering, we generally ask to help. They invariably say, "How do you do it, appearing so comfortable?" Of course, I tell them I can look back at the time I've spent doing it and I tap into what I have learned. I also tell them about how things have not always gone so well and how I tried to treat things as a learning experience.

I remember when I started and was released for the first time to an actual court with actual people and representing an actual person. I was so excited – we often confuse excitement and fear and that was working well for me that day! It was going really well and my case was just about to be called on and then it hit me for the first time. What if I couldn't do it? What if everything I had worked for was finished? Happily, amongst her many talents my mother was a yoga teacher so even back then I knew to take a few breaths and I survived. I achieved the result that was needed and the rest as they say is a career…

Fear of public speaking is widely held to be the foremost fear, even above death. I would suggest there is a way to deal with this fear using the tool of hypnotherapy and NLP. It has fast results, but in general I would suggest small steps. Another way to look at this is to think that you can't do something *yet* – whatever it is, think of small ways to move forward. Finally, the 'power pose'. I cannot tell you how many pupils or coaches, even some who are quite advanced, do this. Prior to interviews and appearances or even before you join a meeting on Zoom, make like Wonder Woman or Superman – put your hands on your hips, which expands the body and take some breaths. The optimum is about two minutes.[6] Whether the science backs it up or not it just works. You may want to do this in a loo or other place where you can't be seen.

Set a goal, use the tools and keep going!

7

HEALTH PILLAR

"Happiness begins with good health."

— DR T. P. CHIA

No trigger warning needed here as the only things I will ask you to look at are things you already do every day: eat, sleep, breathe and move, to see if any minor tweaks (though not running or physical jerks, I promise) you can increase your energy and wellbeing in order to help you feel better and get through your days more easily. It may involve getting up off the sofa a bit more, but no CrossFit, I promise… unless that's what you like.

Where we end in the Permah model is perhaps where we should begin because without this essential ingredient, all the above is more difficult to achieve.

I must start with a disclaimer: I am not a nutritionist, a former professional athlete or a trainer. In the interests of full disclosure, while I once could have been described as having an athletic physique, more than a few years of work stress and life in general have led me to no longer be the little sylph that I was. However, I have always been interested in the topic of health and have read widely. I also know some really great experts who have helped me along the way and have helped me fact check this chapter. Of course, do check with your medics before implementing any of this.

The four pillars to health according to positive psychology (and almost everyone else) are:

Sleep
Nutrition
Movement
Restoration

Let's dive right in.

Sleep – sleep no more... the job, the kiddos, the finances hath murdered sleep... I could go on but you get the picture.

For some, it is a badge of honour that they don't sleep. I know people in my world who don't get much sleep. A lot of my friends are fully paid-up members of the wide-awake club.

Our lifestyles are frantic. We finish our work and family responsibilities late in the night and then reward ourselves with Netflix or doom scrolling. We persuade ourselves that we've earned it because we don't have much time to ourselves. We all know this sort of activity late at night activates parts of our brains that keep us up or, more accurately put, deactivates the thing that puts us to sleep, and yet we do it. This happens in the day too. Studies have shown that while TV or Netflix can be amusing and enjoyable, thereafter you go into a listless, apathetic state and can't move to get those things done that actually would have been fun or at least got you out.

I hate to break it to you: all the studies of the highest performers in the world indicate that it is optimum to eat three hours before bed, stop work two hours before bed, and use no screens an hour before bed. What on earth do people do for the hour! That is the gold standard, of course, but unrealistic for those of us who have work, children and other responsibilities.

There are, however, things you *can* do.

My friends used to joke I was the Margaret Thatcher of sleep (not politically, I hasten to add). She famously slept for four hours a night and that was all she needed. US President Bill Clinton claimed a similar routine. Sadly, Mrs Thatcher developed Alzheimer's and Bill Clinton had to have major heart surgery. There is no evidential link but it seems a bit coincidental. There are a very few who can thrive on very little sleep but they are less than one percent of the population and very few of us are one of those.

THE LAZY GUIDE TOOLS TO MORE OR BETTER SLEEP.

Sleep is the key to wellbeing so what do you do when you can't?

My path to a restful night without counting farm animals began a while ago. One particular night in the wee small hours I was browsing through my phone (absolutely don't do this if sleep is an issue) and I saw a post from a guy called Ali Campbell suggesting hypnosis. I had a session and liked it so much I 'bought the company' (if any of you remember those Remington ads) – well, not the company, but it led to the training and Ali Campbell's mentorship that put me on the path to becoming a clinical hypnotherapist. Hypnotherapy is great for the type of insomnia that wakes you in the middle of the night.

WHAT ELSE CAN YOU DO?

Getting out first thing and exposing your eyes *sans* sunglasses to the light is a well-recognised way of setting your circadian rhythm. Sunlight is optimum but for those of us who live in the UK, light will do. Clearly do not look directly into the sun and protect your eyes if the light is too bright. This is recommended by Andrew Huberman Stanford professor of neurobiology and ophthalmology so he knows.

The other trick is to walk outside during the day. US special forces who have trouble sleeping are prescribed step counters and told to get the steps in. It works for a variety of reasons, not all to do with tiring yourselves out. Those who work with elite athletes also prescribe this so it is worth a go.

Matthew Walker, the world-leading expert on sleep, tells us that if you need to nap during the day, you can, but really not after three pm.

SLEEP HYGIENE

I think it is folklore by now that you remove devices from your bedroom. Blocking out all the light you can with blackout blinds or a sleep mask is also best. Keeping the room cooler helps sleep as does a bath or a shower before bed to regulate your temperature. Reduce the noise. Another good trick is to use a white noise machine or download such an app on your phone – if you have to have it with you then at least it is doing something to assist your sleep. I use a little wind-down myself which I'd like to make available to you as well.

If you can't work the optimum 3:2:1 regime then try this. Try to get the last hour before bed to yourself. If possible, a little before that write down what's bothering you. Get things that are on your mind out – all the stuff that may keep you from sleep. Then give yourself this hour before bed to write a list of things that you must do in the morning so your mind won't have to bother you at three in the morning to remind you to do those things. Finally, before you nod off try to end the day on a positive note by doing the *three good things* exercise priming you to go to sleep on a positive note.

If you wake up in the middle of the night, that may not be as much of a worry as you may think. Apparently, that's what we used to do before the advent of electricity. Try not to get anxious about it. Now is a good time to practise a bit of breathing. Get up for about twenty minutes if you need to and keep the lights low. Maybe read a book, but not a device. Reading is still a kind of resting.

If you are really worn out, I recommend a practice called non-sleep deep rest. It doesn't quite give you all the benefits of sleep but does restore you to a large degree. There is also Yoga Nidra. I have provided you with an audio which may help.

NUTRITION

Please, not another nutrition lecture from someone unqualified to tell you what to do.

We all know what we should do: eat healthily, drink more water, don't eat so many processed foods, eat our greens – those being a little more palatable than back in the day! I think we all would agree with the perceived wisdom of not drinking too much or eating too much fatty, sugary food.

What follows is a decent baseline that not too many people will argue with

THE LAZY GUIDE TOOLS FOR NUTRITION

Whether you're trying to lose weight, fuel for exercise or generally keep healthy, place the emphasis on protein, whichever way you get it. A widely conceived notion is to get between 0.8 and one gram of protein per pound of body weight, whether you are a vegetarian or a meat eater. A palm-sized serving of protein meat or fish is about 23 grams. Half a cup of beans and legumes (about eight grams of protein) is about half the size of your fist. (As a rough guide, a cup is the size of a fist.)

Try to eat about eight hundred grams of fruit and vegetables a day. That is roughly six cups of vegetables/fruit per day. Obviously, a portion of leafy vegetables has to be more than a cup. By filling up on these you will feel less tempted to snack. We all know that vegetables are good for us but there's now research to show that the consumption of vegetables helps with physicality. In a study of females in middle age, taking place over four years, the person who consumed a single serving of vegetables a day was fifty percent more likely to have physical limitations than someone who consumed 2.4 servings.[1] Happily, the fruit and vegetables can come from any source: organic, supermarket, frozen or tinned.

Make that the baseline, and then whatever else you consume you have a healthy foundation. The thinking is that if you fill up on veggies and protein, you're less likely to overdo the rest.

To snack or not to snack, that is the question – what's the answer? If you are hungry, eat. Have a glass of water first to see if you're hungry or just thirsty and then if you need something, eat an apple or similar. If you don't find a piece of fruit or a carrot appealing, maybe you are looking for something more than food. If you need to snack, make sure you have something vaguely healthy about your person.

The rest... to low carb or not to low carb... to fast or not to fast... it is really up to what suits you.

If you like to drink caffeinated beverages (I know there are some odd people who don't), we all have different sensitivities to coffee. You will know where yours lies. As a general rule, no caffeine after two pm is the best I can suggest to my caffeine-loving people out there.

Regarding alcohol, all things in moderation. Here's a tip from my favourite neuroscientist: the dopamine hit you get decreases after the first two sips. Thereafter, the law of diminishing returns applies... and a hangover. One or two drinks is optimal for that reason.

There is so much around sugar addiction and the like at the moment. Of course, limit it, but I also love the suggestion that if you are going to eat sugar, make sure it's in something really good quality, and enjoy it.

There are many devices on the market now which tell you what you need to eat and when. If that is your thing, please do try them out. I think any move to better your health is good.

There are many fitness/calorie trackers if that suits you – I am a fan of MyFitnessPal, where you can enter your food for the day. It also records your fitness activities and gives you a rough estimate of the calories you have used, though a very good tip is not to take the opportunity to eat those extra calories that you have painstakingly burned and stick to the recommended allowance.

I am also currently obsessed with my Oura ring. I made the investment in it as I was fed up of leaving my phone or Fitbit off when I went out for a walk, losing my step count. It is also really interesting when you look at sleep. As I've mentioned, some of those wakeups in the night don't turn out to be as significant as you think when you look at the sleep stats. I am not an affiliate, by the way. I just rate it as a device and it looks pretty too!

WATER, WATER EVERYWHERE

I am like a broken record or whatever the 2023 equivalent of the saying is about drinking a glass of water before you do anything else in the morning. It is related to consistency and being able to hold yourself accountable even when the roof is falling in, but also, what better way to start the day? How much water is enough? If you are thirsty, you haven't drunk enough. Consuming water throughout the day is optimum.

Whenever you feel a little below par in the day, it's a good idea to remind yourself to drink some water. Obviously, if you have pain shooting down your left arm, call a paramedic, but I am sure you get my point.

WHAT ABOUT SUPPLEMENTS?

Of course, the perceived wisdom is you should get all the nutrients you need from your food, but back in the real world that doesn't always happen!

Some supplements are suggested for all of us. Start with Vitamin D. We all need that one, especially those of us who live in a country which has a lot of weather. The UK's NHS website recommends ten micrograms of Vitamin D from September to late March. Omega 3 and a good multivitamin are also suggested for general use.

(If you want to investigate further what may be beneficial to add to your day-to-day regime, I recommend looking at Victoria Health. Their supplements are of the highest quality and their ethics impeccable. Again, I am not an affiliate. I simply rate their products and ethos.)

MOVEMENT

What if there was a pill you could take to make you happier?

It is a trite but true observation that those of us who move more are happier. It is not merely an observation. Moving actually makes you happier.

There is a myriad of things you can do to move your body. The best one for you is the one you like the most, but for those of you who don't like anything other than a slow saunter to the car, here's some information that may help you do what you do already only a tiny bit more. Walking has an impact on our moods and an effect on stress hormones. If something is on your mind, go for a walk. It will dial it down and it apparently also increases our capacity for creative thinking!

THE LAZY GUIDE TOOLS FOR MOVING JUST A LITTLE BIT MORE.

The rules of step club are... there are no rules

Some Japanese marketeers decided that ten thousand steps a day was the thing, a wholly random number that has come into popular culture. This was my baseline through Covid, firstly as a goal to reach incrementally and then to maintain and exceed. It got to the stage that if I hadn't finished my steps in the time allowed, I would do them at home while chatting to a friend in a similar position à la the magnificent Captain Tom as he was before his well-deserved promotion and accolade.

But how many steps should you do? Well, do some and see how you go. The next day do a few more. It is a rare person who doesn't feel any benefit from getting outside and moving. And let me reinforce to you that walking is not an inferior form of exercise. As I've already alluded to, elite special forces are prescribed this, as are top-class NFL and NBA athletes who start training with twenty minutes of walking.

Let's take an example of two women, both 5ft 6 and weighing just over ten stone. One of them burns 101,608 calories a year above her base calories (the number she burns just by doing her day); the other 51,480 extra calories. One of them runs three times a week; one walks five thousand steps a day. Which one burns more calories, do you think? (Heavy hint: this chapter is about steps.)[2] This is amazing to me and I hope to you too. What really moves the needle is inspiring.

You may well have a step counter on your phone and there are a variety of other wearables. I used to get so miffed when I forgot my phone and was out and about walking. If I was doing the steps, I wanted them recorded. As with everything in this book, just noticing and measuring is a really good thing to do.

MINDSET

How about being able to lose weight by doing nothing more than you do already, just by *thinking* it will?

I couldn't not tell you about this amazing study and its results. Eighty-four hotel maids (as they are called in the US), selected from seven different hotels, were split into two groups. All the ladies were reasonably sedentary. Most said they didn't exercise at all and the rest didn't work out regularly. Their weight, measurements and blood pressure were taken at the start of the study.[3]

One group were told that their activities in cleaning the fifteen hotel rooms they did daily met the Surgeon General's recommendation for an active lifestyle. They were told how many calories each activity burned. The other was not told.

A month later the women were spoken to again. The results were remarkable. The group who had been made aware of the guidelines and did no more than they normally would and made no other changes to their lifestyles had lost an average of two lbs each, their blood pressure had dropped by ten points and by all measures the women were significantly healthier and now described themselves as regular exercisers. All expressed a higher degree of satisfaction in their work.

Ellen Langer saw the study as a lesson in mindfulness, which need not involve meditation. She said, "It's about being aware and noticing new things; it's about engagement."

I'll just leave that there for all those who aren't keen on meditation…. hoovering the new Peloton, anybody?

SITTING IS THE NEW SMOKING

While we are talking about getting more movement in the day, I have to mention sitting. During the pandemic lots of us were tied to our chairs and laptops, having meeting after meeting and getting the zoomies.

If you can't get out to walk in the day, just try to stand up more There are certain companies that actually have an in-built pause in their systems so that their employees can get up and move. It certainly helps with sociability and they move more, which is good.

Stand up more often and move around, especially if you've been doing some training. Fidgeting either when sitting or getting up frequently and moving around actually adds to your NEAT (non-exercise activity thermogenesis or calorie burning). People who fidget and get up and move a lot tend to be thinner!

Standing desks are quite the thing and are in some more reconstructed workplaces. When I work from home I improvise and use a chest of drawers as a desk. This is wholly anecdotal but if you've got things like email to do, I find you get a lot more done and are more focused. It doesn't seem to work so well for things you need brain power for. I am writing this sitting down, although allow me to import a tip from my high-performance coaching here. Set a timer for fifty minutes and stop whatever you are doing when the timer goes off. Get up and have a minimum five-minute break to move yourself, and then begin again. Sometimes it can be irritating but it is amazing how much you can get done in that time. This comes from a former world indoor champion procrastinator.

In "Built to Move" Juliet Starett calculated that she burned 275 extra calories using a standing desk during an eight-hour work day. That is the equivalent calorific burn of running twenty-seven marathons in an average work year (260 business days) and this is just by standing up, not even moving. Standing up for eight hours a day is quite a feat (no pun intended) but even scaling it down gives you quite a substantial gain for very little exertion.

LOOK AFTER THOSE PEEPERS

Moving on a little, I thought I'd mention your eyes here. Love or loathe tech, we spend an inordinate amount of time in front of screens. Given this, eye health is becoming increasingly important. Myopia is rife and will be getting worse. A good thing to do is to make sure we simply take regular breaks from the screens, maybe look into the distance when we get up. It is best to do this for two hours a day – split up, of course. I don't think most of us would want to or would get away with staring out the window for two hours at a time. The other is the near/far exercise. Take a pen, hold it at arm's length, and move it closer until you are almost cross-eyed. Then move it away from you. As our eyes get tired and we get older some of us suffer from dry eyes. A really good trick for this is a hot compress.

RESTORATION

By this we mean the time that you take for yourself to wind down. It is an antidote to stress. Again, this is where my fellow trainee coaches and I fell down when I first embarked upon the training. It is something that I have seen a lot in my coaching clients. It is almost as if we get so into the doing of things that we feel to stop would be a waste of time somehow, that we will lose momentum and the never-ending to-do list won't get done. Of course, that is not the case. The opposite is true.

THE LAZY GUIDE TOOLS TO RESTORE YOUR TIRED SELVES

So what to do... sorry, I am going to just say it outright: meditate. An optimum dose is twenty minutes but five minutes will do. You don't even have to sit down; this can be done walking. But the minimum involves just concentrating on breathing in and out for five minutes. If thoughts come to you, notice them as thoughts. If feelings come up, note them as feelings, but let them go.

The other of my absolutes is to take a minute for yourself even during the most hectic of days. Find a quiet place (even if it is in the loo) and close your eyes. Shut out as much as you can and then breathe for one minute. There are many and varied ways of concentrating on the breath, but if you have difficulty with breathing always consult your medical practitioner about the best way for you. People I work with are always surprised by how long a minute feels under those circumstances. When you are being pushed to the max, remember to do this little and often. It can keep you going on your worst days.

OTHER THINGS YOU CAN DO

Get out in nature.
Listen to music.
Savour time to yourself.
Use the audios I have provided as a reset.

COMPOUND YOUR INTEREST

The magnificent success of the British Cycling team was down to their performance coach, Dave Brailsford, who applied the principle of aggregation of marginal gains to the process. This is breaking down the components and increasing everything by just one percent, and repeat. I like to say, keep putting one foot in front of the other, especially when that's all you've got in you to do. Keep plodding on and you'll find your momentum will take you forward. When the momentum builds you may even find you want to do more.

8

RESILIENCE OR HOW TO GROUND YOURSELF WHEN THE GROUND AROUND YOU IS MOVING

"And then resilience enters the room the most elegant of emotional beings, glowing, refined, a reminder that even a flicker of light glows amid the darkness and we can save our tiny ship of troubles from life's stormy seas once again ..."

— SONJA M SWITARTZBACH BSN RN CRN

Here is where we end up! This is the real bonus for paying attention to *happy*. As well as adding happiness to your life and those of the people around us, if you have been able to incorporate any of the suggestions into your daily life then you have a good basis that will keep you centred when 'life' happens.

The events of the last few years have shown our generation that we have resilience. Not in our lifetimes have we been tested in such a way. This natural disaster was non-discriminatory; it didn't happen in some far-off country where we would look on in horror and make donations and then we would forget: it happened to us all. As reasonably well-off people, we are unaccustomed to not truly having control over what happens to us and how we live our lives. I remember hearing years ago, in what now seems a remarkably trivial world event, that the only control we had was the control we had over ourselves. I must have been in one of what I now call my 'resilience-building phases' (ahem) and loudly disagreed with the person on the radio. In my defence, I was stuck in a car on the M25, a challenge for even the most enthusiastic of us. But of course, it is absolutely true and we do. I hope, coming through this book, you know that by doing small things consistently you gain confidence in yourself, and become stronger and happier, and that spreads its benefits to the people with whom we are closest.

Throughout my time in my career, I have marvelled at many people who have managed to overcome the worst of all traumas, and out of that bring something to others who are in the same position. On my wall, I have an example of Kintsugi, a beautiful broken pot mended with gold thread. The Japanese art of repairing broken things with gold, instead of throwing them away makes these things even more beautiful. These people I know – and you may know some too – have found the gold in terrible places and are moving forward, thriving and happy.

To compound the interest of being happy, we can look at what makes a person resilient. It is both interesting and useful to know what makes us resilient. In the field of resilience, it is said that we have to work hard to integrate these things into our lives. I know you are busy being happy. But a little light touch and some awareness can't hurt. You will maybe see a little overlap and be tempted to add in a few of the simpler things. Who wouldn't want to know how to cope better when the ground around you is moving?

What makes a person resilient? Expert researchers on the topic found ten factors.[1]

As coping mechanisms, resilient people...

1. Confronted their fears.
2. Maintained an optimistic but realistic outlook.
3. Sought and accepted social support.
4. Imitated role models.
5. Had their own moral compass.
6. Had some sort of religious or spiritual practice.
7. Attended to their health and wellbeing.
8. Were problem solvers.
9. Looked for meaning and opportunity in the midst of adversity and sometimes even found humour in the middle of the darkness.
10. Accepted to an impressive degree responsibility for their own emotional wellbeing and many used their experiences as a platform for growth.

The people they studied were not all decorated war heroes, although some were. Many would describe themselves as ordinary people who had gone through the darkest times. They didn't immediately bounce back. Many of them had suffered depression, hyper-vigilance and PTSD. The authors were quick to point out that these ten factors were not an exhaustive list but those who took part in the study had described them as crucial or even lifesaving.

How do we create resilience? Well, some of us are naturally better than others – we just are – but that's not to say the rest of us can't learn. We hold the idea that all stress is bad. However, time after time research from a variety of fields shows that there are benefits from the stress response if we learn to manage it.

What I want to emphasise is that there are certain parts of the population who, because of brain injury and significant mental health difficulties, cannot 'bounce back' in the same way as the rest of us. Similarly, there is a section of the population who, due to their lack of basic resources and the security that most of us enjoy, would find this very difficult. For myself, I think it is part of my role going forward to do as much as I can for them in this area and you who are similarly resourced may wish to do that too.

But for those of us who enjoy a certain standard of living, let's do our best to do what we can to make our lives a little more bomb-proof.

REALISTIC OPTIMISM IS KEY TO RESILIENCE

We know now that having and building positive emotions helps enormously with stress. It allows us to step back from the issue and look at it a little more dispassionately. Learning coping mechanisms and new skills means not denying the difficulties but looking for that silver lining. By focusing the attention on the positive and not dwelling on the negative. we can reframe it and look at it in a more positive light so that we can take action that moves us forward.

Martin Seligman describes how pessimists and optimists view past events. Pessimists tend to look at negative events with a sense of permeance. The event stays with them and expands into all areas of life. As an example, if there is a break up of a relationship, pessimists tend to say to themselves that they will never have a good relationship, because partners always behave like... Words you use are very powerful as they focus the mind. Optimists tend to see things as temporary and describe how things have been lately.

So, let's look at four easy ways to bring the sunshine:

1. Focus on what is positive in your life. There will be a lot if you have been noticing the three good things and you can even indulge yourself by looking at happy pics and videos on your phone – those llamas can't help but make you smile!
2. Intentionally think positive thoughts and don't dwell on negative thoughts. I don't mean ignoring all the negative to your detriment, but limiting the negative can mean monitoring our inputs on news and social media. I've noticed anecdotally, certainly as far as crime is concerned, that some of my more obsessed crime fiction lovers and those who follow all the gore on the news are much more convinced of the crime-ridden present rather than my

population who work in the environment all the time.

3. Reframe negative events and interpret them in a more positive way. I don't mean to be trite and when you are in them, just do whatever it takes to look after yourself. But for other less immediate things, know that this won't last forever and take it one day at a time. Use your strengths and see what you can use to deal with the problem and always, *always* notice what is good.

4. Behave in positive ways and take action to build positive feelings. When something is really good and it's down to you, please give yourself some credit for what has happened. I see this so often in my professional life in all sections of the population I coach. It's like… nothing went wrong, great, no mess to clear up, now on to the next. I see this a lot with my clients in the field of medicine. They do not give themselves credit for the enormous amount they contribute in highly straitened circumstances. Behavioural activation, as it's called, is how I got into positive psychology in the first place although I had no idea it was a thing or what it was called. I was just doing what I instinctively thought I needed to, to get through a really difficult time. The idea is that your behaviours affect mood. Too much reinforcement of negative behaviours, crying, talking repetitively about situations and withdrawing from people cause a downward spiral. On the other hand, actively monitoring behaviours by writing them

down and how they made you feel can, over time, lead to an increase in positive feelings. It's good to write down your goals and what you value as they may serve as a motivator to do things that are more helpful for you. After a little time, you may feel like using a journal (or notebook) or planner to put small things in which will help move you towards your goals (and ticking them off as you complete them on a daily basis so you can see how far you have come). Again, please, if you are suffering in any way from depression, the effects of trauma or other mental health issues, please consult your medical practitioner who can best help you.

ARE YOU OPTIMISTIC OR PESSIMISTIC? WHO DO YOU WANT ON YOUR TEAM?

You are the average of the five people you spend most time with so choose them wisely. It's a fact that we can be positively or negatively affected by the moods of the people we spend the majority of our time with. Sometimes we don't have much of a choice about this as they live in our house or we work closely with them. Of course, watch out for the nay-sayers but don't forget to include yourself in that number sometimes. Awareness, again, is key; boundaries are a must but ultimately there are two things to bear in mind. Firstly, you do need the critique and the feedback in your life. Being happy and resilient is not about the emperor's new clothes. If it is incessantly negative and unwarranted you will know and can put your own boundary in place.

Secondly, we all have control over how we feel. You know how to do this and so use what you know.

Following the tools that lead to increased wellbeing and happiness builds you up and it really does have an effect on those around you. See how you go and recharge with the people who truly do bring the joy and the laughs.

ROLE MODELS

Being aware of people and how they affect your life taps into the idea of a role model, certainly as far as the pillars of resilience are concerned. I have spoken before about my father's illness and what I now know was his optimistic response to this. My mother was absolutely inspirational to me in the last months of her life… well, always really. When she, too, survived a heart attack from which she was not supposed to recover, I have an abiding memory of her determined to be up and walking, doing her exercise as she always had done and surprising everyone with how quickly she could move. She had chronic back pain all her life but she sought ways to deal with it through swimming and yoga. She even started a running club and always did her physio and kept active. Those pair are my biggest role models and I try to hold myself to their standard. Every year I do a challenge for them for the British Heart Foundation and notwithstanding my long hours they were always in my mind.

You don't have to know your role models. Back in the day when I was training for an event, I used to come back after a two- and half-hour struggle with the M25 feeling zero interest in going out in the dark, cold and often wet seafront, but it always seemed that on any night when I was going to give myself a bit of a break I would see a lady who was a little advanced in age out for her run, struggling against the weather, really running well. Role model or not, I used to curse her as I struggled up to my flat to change and get out there. She was, however irritatingly, so inspiring and I just felt I had to get out there.

Life is full of inspiring people. I've been following athletes in the Special Olympics (a legitimate and purposeful use of the phone) and have seen some amazing feats of grit and determination: it is quite literally awesome. And yes, I may be sounding a little Pollyanna about it, but it is people like them and their resilience who motivate me when things do not go exactly to plan.

TRAIN YOUR BRAIN

It helps to be on the ball in challenging situations.

A lot of us live our lives in default mode, not really noticing how we get through the day, getting caught up in the doing. Our hard-pressed minds try to cling to the task at hand while dealing with four other things, often at the expense of them all. When we put ourselves completely in the present, we find ourselves better able to deal with more intricate tasks, solve problems and remember quite complicated information. Focus gets lost sometimes so coming back to the here and now helps us with the lack of focus. As I may have mentioned, I'm a great advocate of closing as many tabs literally and figuratively as possible and carving out short periods of time for yourself in a busy day. There are some short audios to help.

NEUROPLASTICITY

So, what about exercises to enhance the brain? Being a life-long learner is associated with a range of health outcomes: wellbeing protection, recovery from mental health difficulties, and an increased capacity to cope with stress-inducing circumstances so well done on reading this... you have increased your wellbeing and resilience, apparently! But we can also do small things. Cathie Hammond University of London Study recommends doing simple things like brushing your teeth or drinking with the 'wrong' hand or getting dressed with your eyes closed. Also playing video games (not to the point of bingeing) is effective too. Whatever activity that is new (and legal) that appeals to you, give it a try.

COMMUNITY - ASK FOR HELP

This is where so many get stuck. Certain jobs and professions lend themselves to a person's desire to keep things to themselves. I'm sure you know some of these people; maybe *you* would never expose what you see as your vulnerability even when you are surrounded by people who would listen. Certain people are categorised as 'the strong one' or the go-to person. Things are changing but slowly for the people who find it the hardest to say how they feel. Often the announcements about wellbeing are in advance of the realities of the day to day.

Part of being resilient is the ability to ask for and give support. This taps again into community. My friend and PT, a former professional boxer, has been very open about his struggles with depression and mental health. He created his own community, espousing and teaching the health components that support resilience, cold water therapies, nutrition and training, of course, but yoga and breath work as well. He, along with many others I have worked with from the military, are role models for speaking out and taking away the sting of vulnerability – a lot of them with a great though somewhat dark sense of humour! (Not that I should have to add this, but that includes female members too.)

EMOTIONAL REGULATION IS ONE OF THE FEATURES OF RESILIENCE AND EVERYDAY DAY LIFE TOO

It consists of two major features when things come up that challenge you. I am not talking about physically dangerous situations here – get out of the situation as quickly and safely as you can.

1. Slowing down – or as I like to call it, *put the lead on the lizard*. Slowing down is putting a little space between you and the issue so you put the brakes on the lizard brain that activates the fight or flight response. Doing that for yourself involves naming

how you feel and experiencing the emotion though not acting on it. At times like this, it is best to get up and move away from the situation if you can. Have a short walk or call a friend. If you can't, then understand you are in a difficult situation and don't say or do the first thing that comes to mind. Try to breathe. There is a space between stimulus and response and that is the place that holds the key to dealing with things.

2. The next part is when you have a little more time to reappraise the situation or thing. What is the emotion telling you? Is it helpful or not? Are there options for you here? Can you make a choice about what you do and do you need information? Wherever you end up, you are making the considered choice.

Working on this helps with cognitive agility which is necessary in navigating our way through the world. We need to be cognitively agile when 'it' hits the fan. We need to have our best way out of there. With a fearful brain it is difficult to see opportunity and a way out, and practising this exercise when things are not quite so acute will help.

SELF-EFFICACY OR SELF-BELIEF AGAIN CAN BE LEARNED AND SHORES UP OUR INNER CONFIDENCE THAT WE CAN OVERCOME THE MOST DIFFICULT OF TIMES

Developing self-efficacy depends on the formula that we have seen so many times during the course of this book, making small steady steps forward. If you have ambitious goals, chunk them down into smaller, achievable goals so you can count your successes along the way. To do away with the all-or-nothing mentality – to falter on one step and then as you've 'failed' not to give up the whole project, learn something from it and keep moving forward getting better and better along the way. Like money compounding, your ability and interest move you forward incrementally in confidence and self-belief until in time there is the tipping point when you achieve that true confidence in yourself.

All of these things build resilience. To be aware of them, to notice them and implement them in your everyday life moves the needle on resilience. Do what you can when you can and as well as you can and you will not fail to increase your resilience quotient and in doing so be the anchor for those around you. There is a gift in being the person in your family, work or friendship on whom people can look for reassurance, stability and grounding. Pollyannish, yes, but with a bit of pride and hopefully a large dollop of humour, for that is a good way of deflecting the negative thoughts which we are taught to have.

Trench humour has its place and has kept many of us going. But don't forget community is there for all of us to ask for and to give help. I would never want it to be like it has been before and hope that shame for vulnerability becomes a thing of the past. Thriving, happy and healthy is your birthright and it's all available to you. You all have these things within you: it's the knowing of it and spending just a little of your precious time on it and you'll be ready to truly enjoy your life and be grounded, should life and the world present you with its next little challenge!

NOW AND NEXT

Thank you so much for taking the time to read this book. I hope it has given you some inspiration and some tools to move things forward. I hope that I have given you a glimpse of how good things can be for you and yours in a life that is lived for the length and the width of it.

I also hope that the end of this book is just the beginning for you and that you want to carry on doing the things that make your life and the lives of those around you lighter and happier. We have only been able to scratch the surface and I hope it will inspire you to do more. And if I can help you along that path, you have my contact details and ways to work with me in the about section.

You do so much for other people that I'd really like it if you took a little time for yourself, but in a nutshell, if you can't do anything else just drink your water, get outside every day and always, always take a minute for yourselves, as many as you can when you can.

With gratitude as ever,

Bev

NOTES

1. WHAT IS HAPPY AND HOW DO YOU GET THERE?

1. Lyubomirsky: *The How of Happiness*
2. For those of you who have younger children (7-12) and teens (12 years plus) whose wellbeing is of concern to you, there are also surveys for them.
3. National Geographic, January 2023
4. All audios can be accessed via the link found at the back of the book

2. POSITIVE EMOTIONS – THE FABULOUS FORTY PERCENT

1. Seligman and Levy at University of Pennsylvania "Authentic happiness" 2002 New York Free Press
2. Fredrickson and Isen: The Value of Positive Emotions. American Scientist 91 330-335
3. All audios can be accessed via the link found at the back of the book
4. 4KWeeks.com
5. Often attributed to Victor Frankel

3. ENGAGEMENT – GO WITH THE FLOW

1. Csikszentmihalyi & Lefevre: "Optimal experiences in work and leisure"
2. All audios can be accessed via the link found at the back of the book
3. All audios can be accessed via the link found at the back of the book,

4. RELATIONSHIPS

1. Barabara Fredrickson
2. Dr Gary Chapman: "5 Love Languages – the secret to love that lasts"

5. MEANING AND PURPOSE – WHY MEANING MATTERS AND WHY WE ALL NEED TO MATTER

1. Robert I Simon: Just a smile and say hello on the Golden Gate Bridge. American Journal Psychiatry
2. Wrzesniewski et al 1997 "Jobs, careers and callings: Peoples relations to their work "Journal of Research in Personality.
3. McQuaid and Kern "Your Wellbeing Blueprint"
4. Audios can be accessed via the link found at the back of the book.
5. Dr Lisa Miller "The Awakened Brain ".

6. ACCOMPLISHMENT – BEING A GOAL-GETTER

1. Levav et al 2011" Extraneous factors in judicial decisions"
2. Unattributed from website Peaceful Mind, Peaceful Life
3. Charles Snyder
4. Audio link at the back of the book
5. Sonja Lyubomirsky – The How of Happiness
6. Amy Cuddy Ted Talk "Your body language may shape who you are "

7. HEALTH PILLAR

1. Built to Move Kelly and Juliet Starett
2. Doctor Kelly and Juliet Starrett: "Built to Move"
3. Crum and Langer: Mindset Matter Exercise and the new placebo effect. Psychological Science 18 no 2

8. RESILIENCE OR HOW TO GROUND YOURSELF WHEN THE GROUND AROUND YOU IS MOVING

1. Charnley and Southwick Resilience

ACKNOWLEDGMENTS

This has been an absolute treat to write as I have been able to think about and thank all of the people who have been so significant in my life and to a greater or not much lesser degree made me the person I am today. The list is long but please indulge me. I have a lot to be grateful for (and it'll save me writing a lot of gratitude letters).

To Mum and Dad, my heroes and inspiration, I owe it all to you.

To Phil, my little brother, who is one the funniest and kindest people I know, and H sis-in-law though sister really, thank you, thank you for everything including the mint Aero.

To Ellie, Rhys and Jac, you are all my favourites.

To my other mother Deryn and "sister" Jane and all of you at Beryl Road, what an amazing way to grow up.

To Dawn Aloof, miss you always and our adventures together, hope you have found your calm waters.

To Penny Jenks and Penny Muir, apparently, you can only be my besties if you are called Penny. Thank you for your support, inspiration and laughs. And you too, of course, Deb, the exception that proves the rule.

To the cousins' congress, loves you all and thank you for propping me up and to Yvette, you're my favourite unicorn.

To Kev my other 'brother', much loved by Dot and John, for being by my side at some of the most difficult times of my life, for Polperro and those caring compassionate kicks up the backside you deliver every now and again, motivation at its finest!

To Katrina, yet another "sibling" loved by Dot and John, we wuz wild then and wear knitwear now: so glad we are still in each other's lives.

To the Barry babes at home and abroad, what an amazing bunch you all are!

To Bozzie and all my law girls and boys, my tribe we've kept each other going over the years and are all still here to tell the tale.

To our Hoffie gang and my darling Kate, such an amazing time, so glad I spent it with you and remembering our dear Bob.

To Iain Jacko Jackson for getting up very early and training me when you knew I was stuck at court. Thank you for all your wise advice on all thing's fitness, being a sounding board and a really good laugh.

To Bhavna such a talent and shining light in medicine, who always brings the glam and Fiona for her unfailingly funny take on absolutely everything: glad you're in my life.

To my mentor's past and present: Ali Campbell, who introduced me to an amazing new world and never fails to put me to sleep. To Carol Deveney, for your wisdom, the laughs and for giving up your time to beta-read this book.

To Lisa Johnson who understood, "you just want to make people happy". To Niyc Pigeon, so grateful for opening up the amazing world of positive psychology for me. To Abigail Horne and Deanne Adams, passionate book lovers and superb wordsmiths, thank you, and to Carol and Matt at Authors and Co for this amazing book cover and all your very patient help with the book.

And to all my new tribe who I've met in my new career, thank you all so much for your support and the laughs: Antoinette, Kim, Maria "STBS" Anderson, Fiona, Tom, Nic, Liz, Karen, Graham and Zara and so many more. Really looking forward to spending more time with you and seeing how this exciting new future is going to unfold.

And finally, and it really is finally, to all the people I've met over the years who I can't name. Your strength and resilience continue to inspire me and are at the heart of all I do.

ABOUT THE AUTHOR

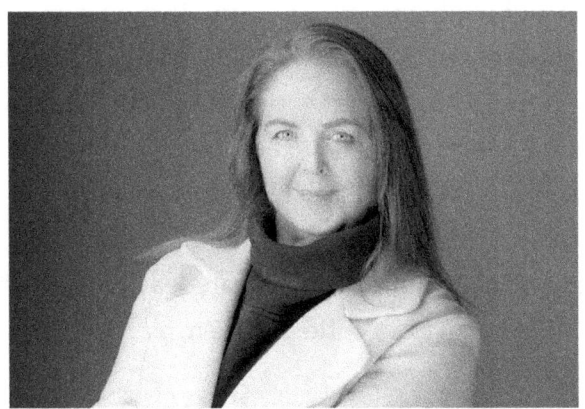

BEV CRIPPS

Bev is a barrister and this year sees her thirty-fifth anniversary of being called to the bar, practising in the criminal courts of England and Wales and also Courts Martial.

She set up her coaching company BCConnection Ltd in 2020 to, as she puts it, "help people in a different way". She is a qualified clinical hypnotherapist, positive psychology coach and licentiate resilience trainer. An accomplished and entertaining speaker, Bev has delivered training both to solicitors and barristers, police and, more latterly, in the NHS.

She has a trademarked coaching system Reset, Rewire Resilience®, a twelve-week bespoke private coaching course, the fundamentals of which you will find in this book. She delivers resilience and positive psychology training both for companies and coaches. Her Reset package of Hypnotherapy and/or NLP deals with any issues that are holding you back such as phobias, weight loss, or anxiety.

Bev was adopted and brought up by amazing parents, though throughout her working life she has been acutely aware of how fate can dictate how one's path in life goes and that she could very easily have become one of the children in care whom she so often saw as clients or victims of crime because of their circumstances. With that in mind, her intention is to set up a foundation for care leavers in memory of her parents to provide a little of the support that she was so lucky to have had.

Bev grew up by the sea in Barry and is a proud Welsh woman who emigrated and now lives by the sea in England.

CONNECT WITH ME

Link for the bonus audios is at
https://mybcconnection.com/book/

For interviews, speaking engagements/speaker bio or comment opportunities please contact:
gethelp@mybcconnection.com or
www.mybcconnection.com

You will find me on:
Facebook.com/BCConnection
Facebook.com/Get Conscious with the Connection - Free Facebook Community.
Instagram.com/bc_connection1
Linkedin.com/Bev Cripps

www.ingramcontent.com/pod-product-compliance
Lightning Source LLC
Chambersburg PA
CBHW060104230426
43661CB00033B/1410/J